T0192024

Lecture Notes of the Institute for Computer Sciences, Social Informatics and Telecommunications Engineering 432

More information about this series at https://link.springer.com/bookseries/8197

Susanna Spinsante · Bruno Silva ·
Rossitza Goleva (Eds.)

IoT Technologies for Health Care

8th EAI International Conference, HealthyIoT 2021
Virtual Event, November 24–26, 2021
Proceedings

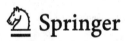 Springer

Editors
Susanna Spinsante 🄳
Marche Polytechnic University
Ancona, Italy

Bruno Silva 🄳
University of Lisbon
Lisbon, Portugal

Rossitza Goleva 🄳
New Bulgarian University
Sofia, Bulgaria

ISSN 1867-8211 ISSN 1867-822X (electronic)
Lecture Notes of the Institute for Computer Sciences, Social Informatics
and Telecommunications Engineering
ISBN 978-3-030-99196-8 ISBN 978-3-030-99197-5 (eBook)
https://doi.org/10.1007/978-3-030-99197-5

This Springer imprint is published by the registered company Springer Nature Switzerland AG
The registered company address is: Gewerbestrasse 11, 6330 Cham, Switzerland

Preface

We are delighted to introduce the proceedings of the eighth edition of the European Alliance for Innovation (EAI) International Conference on IoT Technologies for Health-Care (HealthyIoT 2021). This conference brought together researchers, developers, and practitioners around the world who are contributing towards the design, development, and deployment of healthcare solutions based on IoT technologies, standards, and procedures. This year the emphasis has been on using IoT to respond to epidemic/pandemic situations and on the security aspects – keeping the critical IoT infrastructure safe and running in states of emergency.

The technical program of HealthyIoT 2021 consisted of 17 full papers, including one invited paper, in oral presentation sessions at the conference tracks. Oral sessions included high-quality technical presentations of the papers submitted to the HealthyIoT 2021 track, but also of those papers submitted to two other tracks, namely "Wearables in Healthcare" and "AI-assisted Solutions for COVID-19 and Biomedical Applications in Smart Cities", both of which consisted of two oral presentations.

Coordination with the steering chair, Imrich Chlamtac, was essential for the success of the conference. We sincerely appreciate his constant support and guidance. It was also a great pleasure to work with such an excellent organizing committee team for their hard work in organizing and supporting the conference. In particular, we are grateful to the Technical Program Committee who completed the peer-review process or technical papers and helped to put together a high-quality technical program. We are also grateful to the Conference Manager, Elena Davydova, for her support and all the authors who submitted their papers to the HealthyIoT 2021 conference.

We strongly believe that the HealthyIoT conference provides a good forum for all researchers, developers, and practitioners to discuss all science and technology aspects that are relevant to the creation of healthcare solutions based on IoT technologies, standards, and procedures. We also expect that the future HealthyIoT conferences will be as successful and stimulating as this year's, as indicated by the contributions presented in this volume.

February 2022

Susanna Spinsante
Bruno Silva
Rossitza Ivanova Goleva
Ivan Miguel Serrano Pires
Petre Lameski
Eftim Zdravevski

Organization

Steering Committee

Imrich Chlamtac   University of Trento, Italy

Organizing Committee

General Chair

Susanna Spinsante   Università Politecnica delle Marche, Italy

General Co-chairs

Bruno Silva   Universidade Europeia and Universidade da Beira Interior, Portugal

Rossitza Ivanova Goleva   New Bulgarian University, Bulgaria

Technical Program Committee Co-chairs

Ivan Miguel Serrano Pires   Instituto Politécnico de Viseu, Portugal

Petre Lameski   University of Ss. Cyril and Methodius in Skopje, Macedonia

Eftim Zdravevski   University of Ss. Cyril and Methodius in Skopje, Macedonia

Sponsorship and Exhibit Chair

Nuno M. Garcia   Universidade da Beira Interior, Portugal

Workshops Chair

Nuno Cruz Garcia   Universidade de Lisboa, Portugal

Publicity and Social Media Chair

Angelica Poli   Università Politecnica delle Marche, Italy

Publications Chair

Aleksandar Jevremovic   Singidunum University, Serbia

Web Chair

Gonçalo Marques   Polytechnic of Coimbra, Portugal

Technical Program Committee

Alessia Paglialonga	National Research Council (CNR), Italy
An Braeken	Vrije Universiteit Brussel, Belgium
Marko Sarac	Singidunum University, Serbia
Sandeep Pirbhulal	Norwegian University of Science and Technology, Norway
Virginie Felizardo	Universidade da Beira Interior, Portugal
Ivan Ganchev	University of Limerick, Ireland
Ennio Gambi	Università Politecnica delle Marche, Italy
Emmanuel Conchon	University of Limoges, France

Contents

Security and Privacy - Software and Application Security

Non-intrusive and Privacy Preserving Activity Recognition System for Infants Exploiting Smart Toys

Niko Bonomi and Michela Papandrea$^{(\boxtimes)}$

University of Applied Sciences and Arts of Southern Switzerland (SUPSI),
Lugano, Switzerland
{niko.bonomi,michela.papandrea}@supsi.ch

Abstract. The Human Activity Recognition (HAR) research area showed great advances in the last decade, achieving excellent prediction performances and great applicability, which is reflected on the wearable sensors market adoption. However, most of the research effort concentrated on an adult target population. When considering a younger population of infants or children, currently available HAR solution based on wearable devices are not applicable anymore. In this paper we present an HAR based solution targeting infants, based on a non-intrusive and privacy-preserving measurement methodology which allows the preservation of children behaviour and the collection of objective data (particularly important for clinical observation purposes). The proposed solution, based on the usage of a set of smart toys (AutoPlay toys-set) achieves great performances in the recognition of a set of 12 toy-activity pairs, reaching accuracy values up to 96%. These results pave the way to a broad application of the presented methodology on objective analysis of humans motor skills.

Keywords: Activity · Motricity · Infants · Neurodevelopment · Toys · HAR · Infants activity recognition

1 Introduction

In the last decade, thanks to the miniaturization of hardware components, it has been quite easy to equip almost every digital device with some sort of sensors and actuators that coupled with transmission capabilities enable an endless number of possibilities. One of such possibility is Human activity recognition (HAR), which nowadays is widespread in everyday objects, like smartwatches or fit-tracker. HAR main goal is to identify and interpret the actions executed by a human based on some measured sensor data. HAR can be performed using information coming from different sources like smartphone or wearable sensors, camera footage, LIDAR technology: those observations are feed to an intelligent algorithm that performs a prediction based on supervised knowledge.

© ICST Institute for Computer Sciences, Social Informatics and Telecommunications Engineering 2022
Published by Springer Nature Switzerland AG 2022. All Rights Reserved
S. Spinsante et al. (Eds.): HealthyIoT 2021, LNICST 432, pp. 3–18, 2022.
https://doi.org/10.1007/978-3-030-99197-5_1

The HAR research area showed great advances in the last decade, achieving excellent prediction performances and great applicability, which is reflected by the growth of the wearable sensors marked. However, most of the research effort concentrated on the adult target population. When considering a younger population of infants or children, currently available HAR solutions based on wearable devices are not applicable anymore [7]. Wearable sensors introduce a bias in the young Human Activity Recognition (yHAR) systems: children tend to focus their attention on the sensor device itself hence their behavior is not natural. Solutions based on cameras recordings are adopted instead, reaching not very accurate results on very small children (i.e., infant skeleton extraction from videos is still a challenge) and dealing with the issue of privacy.

AutoPlay [4] is an innovative project which deals with the challenges of young Human Activity Recognition: it adopts the aforementioned HAR technologies in the field of infants neuro-development monitoring. The AutoPlay general goal is to anticipate the diagnosis of autism spectrum disorders (ASD), neuro developmental disorders and other social fragilities. The AutoPlay methodology is based on a toys kit, a set of smart toys equipped with sensors, for infants motor skills interpretation. The sensors allow the collection of inertial data (e.g., accelerometer, gyroscope and magnetometer). The usage of such smart-toys provides an effective measurement methodology when applied to very small children: this is to handle the important issue present when dealing with the measurement of motricity of children which are very small, or very sensitive at a sensory perception level. It does not provide an obstacle to the freedom of movement when compared to bulky wearable sensors. And, additionally, it does not affect the privacy of small infants, as opposed to video recording and computer vision based methodologies. In this paper we present the results of applying current HAR methodologies exploiting the AutoPlay smart toys, as non-worn sensors.

The results obtained and presented in this work are encouraging and demonstrating that nowadays available technology is ready for such application, paving the way for a broad adoption of non intrusive and privacy preserving methodologies for the observation and monitoring of infants, and more in general for fine motor-skills measurement.

In this paper we provide a brief description of the related SoA (Sect. 2). Successively, Sect. 3 describes the methodologies we exploited to collect training data for the predictive models. In Sect. 4 we describe the learning approach and, finally, in Sect. 5 we describe the obtained results, distinguishing between in-lab and real use-case scenarios.

2   Related Work

Nowadays, human activity recognition (HAR) services are embedded in almost every wearable smart devices (e.g., smart watches, fitness trackers, etc.) and companion devices such as smartphones. The main objective of such embedded HAR services is the identification of humans movements and actions, and the recognition of behavioral patterns on the base of heterogeneous measured data.

There exist various types of wearable sensors, meant for being worn on different parts of the human body. Those kinds of sensors might be uncomfortable to be worn, this means that they are not a good solution for long term monitoring of human activities. In the last decade the smartphone industry evolved, allowing the embedding of those kinds of sensors directly on a portable device that almost everybody carries in their pocket. This kind of sensors bring up new research opportunities for human-centered activity recognition. They usually embed three axis accelerometer, gyroscope, microphone, camera and many more sensors depending on the vendor. Nowadays almost every smartphone is equipped with such sensors that coupled with smart algorithms provide the user useful information such as the daily amount of steps, workout session duration and also some more interesting metrics like the sleep quality.

From the related literature, Anguita et al. [1] collected and shared a dataset of human activities from various persons and annotated in each time unit the activity that the person was carrying out: this allowed the generation of a ground truth where the data is connected to a human activity. The generated dataset contains accelerometer and gyroscopic sensors data collected from smartphones. Exploiting this dataset they have trained a support vector machine classifier using a rolling window of about 2 s and a step of 50% of the size of the window, and achieved an activity prediction accuracy score of 74%. Also Papandrea et al. [6] have applied such methodology in a location prediction and mobility modelling system, with the main goal of cutting computational costs and increasing the prediction performances based on a personalization strategy. Also in this case they have applied an averaging moving window to compute the necessary features, and reached an accuracy score of 94% in the prediction of 9 different activities.

The research study presented in this paper concerns the HAR methodologies applied to toddlers, and more in particular with the support of augmented toys. Numerous works in literature have already exploited this topic, Rivera et al. [7] presented an architecture of augmented toys, consisting of smart cubes that are able, using a set of light sensors, to detect how they are oriented and how they are placed with respect to other cubes. They share the observation related to the issue of children wearing conventional wearable sensors, stating that this could alter children behaviour and cause distractions, thus invalidating the measurements. This is actually the main reasons behind the practice of embedding sensors inside common objects, like toys, so that the children are not disturbed and biased by them.

An interesting work carried out by T. L. Westeyn et al. [11] in 2010, presents a toys-kit that helps in the annotation process of children activities trough cameras and sensors embedded within toys. The author proposed a specific tool that exploits smart toys as an assistant to a video-monitoring system for children and adults. They presented good results obtained on the gathered data, performing a support vector machine based classification to classify the kind of activity played by the child (i.e., jumps, shake, spin etc.).

Many different Inertial Measurement Units sensors are available on the market at affordable prices, and with an acceptable measurement resolution for HAR application. Among these, the Shimmer IMU is a sensor device widely exploited among different research projects, especially medical applications. Mehmood et al. [5] exploited this sensor in the field of human activity recognition. They have obtained some encouraging results with sampling frequency 50 Hz, demonstrating it allows the collection of all relevant information about human activities. Using a wide set of classification algorithms they have discovered that the *support vector machine* performs very well for the recognition of stationary activities like sit, lying down, stand still, etc., meanwhile the *random forest* algorithm reaches great results on non-static activities recognition like running, walking, jumping etc. In the field of activity recognition, an interesting work has been carried out by [2] Antar et al.; it showcases the challenges in the field of HAR based on wearable sensors, providing a complete description on how to perform an initial Exploratory Data Analysis (EDA), on which filters needs to be used during the preprocessing phase, on how to perform an effective segmentation of the data and on which are the features that are worth considering in the case that the data will be feed into an intelligent algorithm.

With this paper we intend to advance the current SoA presenting the application of supervised technologies to a more challenging research problem, the *indirect infant activity recognition*. With the proposed approach we aim to provide new tools to the infants and childhood health research area, more specifically with the goal of anticipating ASD diagnosis.

3   The Dataset

A set of measurement sessions have been carried out to sample inertial data: each measurement consists in a play session exploiting the AutoPlay toys kit [4] and collects a 9-dimentional raw dataset consisting of *3D acceleration low noise, 3D acceleration wide range* and *3D gyroscope data* . Each toy is tailored to accommodate one or more IMU sensors.

The sensor node of choice is the Shimmer IMU unit which is equipped with multiple sensors: low-noise and wide range accelerometer, gyroscope, magnetometer, humidity and temperature sensor and altimeter, allowing to sample data at a frequency up to 2048 samples per second [9].

The measurement sessions have been enriched with the help of cameras that enable the annotation of the activities carried out by the human, thus allowing to create a supervised dataset for the training of activity prediction algorithms. The cameras recorded videos at 25 fps: the synchronization between the collected data and the recorded videos have been performed with a two-phases synchronization methodology, presented in [8]. Each session was manually post processed in order to associate a ground truth to the data: each frame of a video is associated with an activity, and each sample of the collected data is associated to a frame (hence to an activity as well).

3.1   Synthetic Dataset: In-Lab Data Collection

A first dataset was collected directly in lab, allowing for an easy data acquisition process necessary to create a labeled training dataset.

The dataset includes samples related to three toys: an elephant, a small ball and a car (Fig. 1). The elephant and the ball had one sensor node mounted inside the toy, meanwhile the car has two sensors mounted directly into two wheels (one in the front, one in the back of the car) allowing the independent measurement of both front and rear wheels movements.

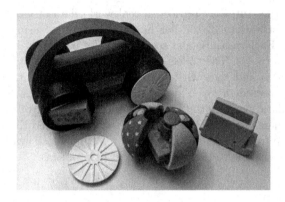

Fig. 1. Toys used in lab

The dataset contains a set of (different) activities per toy. In total we collected samples belonging to 12 different couples <toy, activity> (list of activities per toy is reported in Table 1). The listed activities have been identified to be the most representative ones for toddler (9–24 months) in terms of frequency of appearance, as observed during a real world data gathering sessions involving children. Our goal was to select a reduced set of significant activities, which are interesting from an activity recognition point of view, and feasibly implementable in a more realistic scenario.

Table 1. Toys activities

Car	Ball	Elephant
Drive	Toss	Let it fall
Overturn	Roll over	Overturn
Turn wheel	Shake	Throw
Knock	Turn	Knock

The in-lab data collection involved two adult persons: each of them performed a data collection session of 7 min for each pair <toy, activity>. This resulted in a total of 168 min of data collected in lab for the synthetic settings.

An additional synthetic data measurement session was performed to sample a mixed sequence of activities, where each involved person simulated the movements of a toddler playing with the exploited toys. Each person had the possibility to freely choose the amount of time to dedicate to each activity (in the list shown above) and the order of the activities in the sequence. This resulted in a total amount of 12 min of collected data.

3.2   The AutoPlay Dataset

In the scope of the AutoPlay project, a real world dataset has been gathered. Data from a vast variety of toddler have been sampled using the AutoPlay augmented toys. Each measurement session has also been recorded with cameras for annotation purposes. The collected sensor data has been synchronized with the captured video and thus with the annotated ground truth thanks to the methodology presented in [8]. This work proposed an approach for two main problems: the data synchronization issue, due to the lack of synchronization between the cameras used to record the toddler playing and the actual sensors installed into the toys (without an on-board real time clock available), and the data-time alignment due to the sensor clock drift problems.

3.3   Annotation

The annotation procedure have been possible thanks to the footage captured by various cameras installed on the measurement environment. Each video is then post-processed manually and each frame of the video is associated with an activity declared in a specific pool of possible activities selected a priori. In the case of the in-lab data acquisition this pool of possible activities was reduced to 4 per each toy (as mentioned above) meanwhile the AutoPlay dataset is comprehensive of a large set of defined activities which can be categorized in macro groups.

- **Functional**: A functional activity is described as an activity that can enable another subsequent set of activities. The functional activity is used to achieve an objective such as stack some toys to build a tower or push away a non desired toy.
- **Exploratory**: An exploratory activity allows, as suggested by the term, the toddler to explore both the environment and the toys properties stimulating the 5 senses.
- **Rotation**: This is a category of activities in which the toddler performs some kind of rotation of the toy with an exploitative purpose, of as a functional activity.

Table 2 shows the complete list of possible activities identified for the Auto-Play dataset.

Table 2. Complete list of infants play activity of reference

Activity	Category
Push	Functional
Shift	Functional
Lay	Functional
Lift	Functional
Lower	Functional
Drag	Functional
Throw	Functional
Tender	Functional
Grab	Functional
Knock over	Functional
Stack	Functional
Pick	Exploratory
Hold in hand	Exploratory
Let it fall	Exploratory
Shake	Exploratory
Hit	Exploratory
Bite	Exploratory
Knock	Exploratory
Turn	Rotation
Overturn	Rotation
Roll over	Rotation

4   Predictive System

In order to build a predictive methodology able to identify, given raw inertial data (as described in Sect. 3), the related toddler activity we realized a data workflow which includes the following steps:

1. data collection (described in Sect. 3)
2. data annotation (described in Sect. 3.3);
3. data synchronization (as described in [8]);
4. features extraction;
5. activity prediction model training and parameter tuning;
6. model validation on real use-case data.

Regarding the *features extraction* phase (point 4 of the workflow), we calculated a feature vector of 14 variables per each dimension of the input raw data, including standard statistical features like: mean, standard deviation, max, min and signal vector amplitude (as presented in [1]).

Table 3. Feature vector of 14 variables calculated per each raw input data dimension

Feature	Description
min	Min value
max	Max value
mean	Signal mean
mad	Median absolute value
std	Standard deviation
pow	Signal power
skew	Skewness
kurtosis	Kurtosis
deriv mean	mean of the derivative
deriv std	Standard deviation of the derivative
SMA	Signal magnitude area
entropy	Signal entropy
iqr	Interquartile range
snr	Signal to noise ratio

The 9-dimentional raw data (acceleration low noise 3DoF, acceleration wide range 3DoF, giroscope 3DoF) is enriched with the *magnitude* of the acceleration vector, generating a 10-dimensional features vector. Among the 14 variables shown in Table 3, only 13 of them are calculated over all the 10 raw dimensions. The SMA variable is computed using Eq. 1 over the 3-dimensional axis of the acceleration low noise. Hence the final resulting features vectors belong to a 131-dimensional space.

$$SMA = \frac{\sum_{n=1}^{N_x} |x_n| + \sum_{n=1}^{N_y} |y_n| + \sum_{n=1}^{N_z} |z_n|}{N_{samples}} \tag{1}$$

The features described above have been calculated per each raw sample data. As part of the features extraction phase, we calculated the features over a temporal window. In order to generate the training set for our activity prediction model we extracted aggregated features over the above mentioned temporal window, sliding it over time; in particular the window is sliding over the temporal signal of a fixed sized step. In the following sections we describe the study performed in order to identify the optimal values for both *window size* and *sliding step length*. The objective of this study is to find the smallest possible windows size and step length necessary to carry detailed information about the activity performed, without compromising the performances of the activity recognition classifier. The objective related to the size of the window, is driven by the necessity of being responsive in the recognition of the activity, in a context where the mean duration of an activity is the order of seconds.

In the first instance we performed a grid search for the window size optimal value, fixing the sliding step length to 25% of the window. The metric used to evaluate the performances of the activity classification model per each window size value, is the *accuracy*. This procedure has been performed separately per each toy, because the average infant activity duration strictly depend on the exploited toy.

For what concern the **ball** toy, as shown in Fig. 2a, the best window size obtained is identified by the global maximum of the window size versus accuracy graph, in the searched range: the optimal value found correspond to 100 samples, that means 1 s window size.

Fixing a window size value of 100 sample, we performed a grid search for the optimal value of the sliding step length. Figure 2b shows a scatter plot representing the results of the search. As visible from the graph, searching in a range [10–40]% of the window size, we get similar results in fact all the accuracy values associated with the different sliding sizes resulted in a model accuracy of approximately 95.5%. We decided to pick a reasonably small value in the search

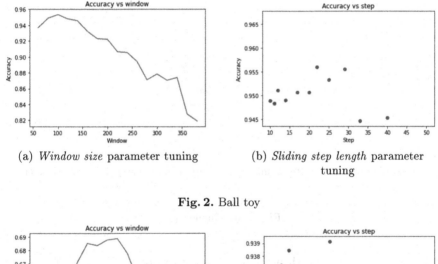

(a) *Window size* parameter tuning

(b) *Sliding step length* parameter tuning

Fig. 2. Ball toy

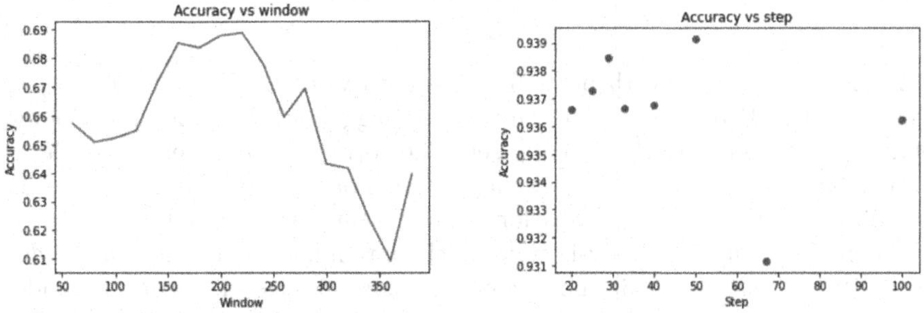

(a) *Window size* parameter tuning

(b) *Sliding step length* parameter tuning

Fig. 3. Car toy

range (step size length = 20 samples, that is 20% of the window size), which allowed both to avoid overfitting and to have a consistent training dataset, at the same time. Summarizing, the procedure has identified an optimal window size of 100 samples (1 s) and an overlay step of 20 samples (0.2 s).

The same process has been performed with the **car** toy related data (Fig. 3a). In this case the identified optimal window size corresponds to 220 samples (2.2 s). Also in this case we plotted (Fig. 3b) the activity prediction accuracy versus the sliding step size: there is no clear trend in the plot, considering a search range of [20–100] samples. The related accuracy ranges from 93.1% to 93.9%: we have selected 50 samples as optimal step, because it is producing the highest accuracy score.

For what concerns the **elephant** toy, Fig. 4a shows the plot of accuracy vs window size. We have selected the optimal window size located on the global maximum of the range, more precisely at a window size of 260 (2.6 s) samples. As we can observe in Fig. 4b, the accuracy does not show a clear trend in correlation with the sliding step length, and it floats around the value 70.5%. A sliding step size of 60 samples (0.6 s) has been selected.

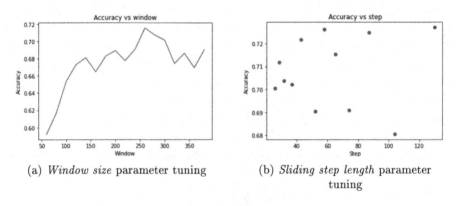

(a) *Window size* parameter tuning

(b) *Sliding step length* parameter tuning

Fig. 4. Elephant toy

In order to proceed with point 5 in the data workflow (*model training*) we calculated the 131-dimensional features vectors aggregating on the time windows defined above, to create the training set. The correlation between the obtained features has been calculated. No particular cases of high correlated features has been observed: the highest correlation value obtained is around 40%.

We proceed with the analysis training three well known classifiers: a *random forest* [10], an *ada boost* [3] and a *gradient boost* [3] classifier. For the models parameters tuning we performed a grid search over multiple parameters values ranges, in order to find the best parameters values. We adopted an 8-fold stratified cross validation to assess the performances of the trained model, averaging on the *accuracy* per each fold.

5   Results

5.1   Results Based on the In-Lab Collected Dataset

As stated above, the dataset collected in lab and described in Sect. 3 was divided into two sets: using the 80% for the training phase and the remaining 20% for testing. From the selected possible classifiers mentioned in Sect. 4, we selected the *Gradient Boost* to be the best performing one. The tables presented below show the performances of the classifier trained separately on each of the toy-related dataset. In all the three cases, the trained classification models show very good performances.

Ball. As shown in Table 4, the classification model trained on the ball related dataset has good performances. The values reported have been calculated over a test set where the activity classes are balanced (as it is on the training set), after the parameters tuning phase. As it is possible to observe in the classification report, the accuracy is quite high with an average value of 97% on the in-lab collected test set.

Table 4. Ball in-lab dataset based classification report

	Precision	Recall	F1-score	Support
Throw	1.00	0.99	0.99	774
Roll over	0.92	1.00	0.96	774
Shake	1.00	0.92	0.96	774
Turn	0.99	0.99	0.99	774
Accuracy			0.97	3096
Macro avg	0.98	0.97	0.97	3096
Weighed avg	0.98	0.97	0.97	3096

Elephant. Similarly, also the classifier trained over the elephant related dataset performs very well (Table 5): also in this case the test average accuracy is 97%.

Car. Is worth noting that the car-data based classifier is performing slightly worse compared to the previously presented ones (performances shown in Table 6). This is mainly due to the fact that the classifier shows difficulties in distinguishing between the activities *turning wheel* and *slide*. This is mainly due to the fact that this toy, as in its lab configuration, has a single sensor node located inside a back wheel. In the case of *turning wheel* activity, the kid is turning the wheels with one hand, while holding the car with the other hand. Meanwhile the *slide* activity is performed by make the car wheels rolling on the ground. The resulting signal sampled by the sensors show only slight differences between the

Table 5. Elephant in-lab dataset based classification report

	Precision	Recall	F1-score	Support
Let it fall	0.98	0.95	0.96	220
Overturn	0.96	0.95	0.96	220
Knock	0.96	0.99	0.98	220
Throw	0.98	0.99	0.98	220
Accuracy			0.97	880
Macro avg	0.97	0.97	0.97	880
Weighed avg	0.97	0.97	0.97	880

two actions. The solution adopted for this problem is to install two sensor nodes in the car, one in a front wheel and the other in a rear wheel. With this sensors configuration, we distinguish the turning wheel activity from the sliding activity (where both wheels roll at approximately the same rate): this configuration has been exploited in the real world use-case sampling sessions.

Table 6. Car in-lab dataset based classification report

	Precision	Recall	F1-score	Support
Slide	0.99	0.91	0.95	296
Overturn	0.98	0.93	0.95	296
Knock	0.94	0.98	0.96	296
Turning wheels	0.91	0.99	0.95	296
Accuracy			0.95	1184
Macro avg	0.95	0.95	0.95	1184
Weighed avg	0.95	0.95	0.95	1184

5.2   Validation of the In-Lab Data Base Classification Models

To asses the performances of the models trained over the in-lab collected data, it is important to perform a validation, which allows us to measure how well the proposed methodology is able to generalise: this is carried out exploiting an additional in-lab collected dataset, which the models have never seen before, and assessing the related performance. This validation step concerning in-lab data, has been carried out on data collected by two adult people (a man and a woman), which freely played with the AutoPlay toys, performing autonomously sequences of activities from the list of predefined ones, selected per each specific toy (see Sect. 3).

Table 7. Validation over in-lab collected data

Toy	Precision	Recall	F1-score	Accuracy
Car	0.84	0.71	0.70	0.71
Ball	0.96	0.96	0.96	0.96
Elephant	0.73	0.73	0.70	0.71

Table 7 shows the performances measured during this validation phase: it shows that the trained models achieve good classification performances both in terms of precision, recall, F1-score and accuracy. The *ball* related activity classification shows the best results, achieving 96% of accuracy (weighted average per activity). The *elephant* and *car* related activity classification experiences lower accuracy scores of 71%: however, given the hardness of the classification task, due to the peculiarity and noise of the activities, we could consider the achieved score to be acceptable. The main problem associated with the car related classification, as mentioned in the previous section, reseeds in the fact that it wrongly predict the 'slide' activity as 'turning wheel' activity. Regarding the elephant toy, on this validation phase, the trained model locates most of its prediction error for the activity 'Trow', which is interpreted erroneously as 'Knock': this is because a part of the 'Trow' activity includes a phase in which the elephant toy hits the ground, and in terms of forces acting on the toy and measured by the accelerometer these are similar to the ones measured during the 'Knock' activity. A dynamical window size approach could eventually mitigate this issue.

5.3 Validation on Real Use-Case Scenarios

In order to evaluate the performances of the proposed models on a real use case scenario involving children, we performed a second validation phase. This includes data collected from real world experiments involving small children (average target age is 2 years old). For the data collection, the AutoPlay complete toy set is provided to 3 children, which independently and autonomously play with them, without any request from or interaction with an adult person. The children are observed and data is collected through embedded sensors and cameras, as for the in-lab measurements described above. The complete data collected correspond to approximately 30 min of measurement. The measurement environment is shown in Fig. 5.

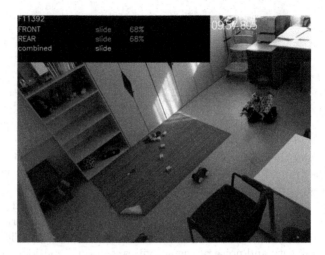

Fig. 5. Real use-case scenario: measurement environment

The results obtained by feeding the collected data to the models trained with the in-lab scenario data, show promising performances. The trained models are performing very well in recognizing rotation related activities (i.e., reaching 79% accuracy on ball 'roll-over' prediction, and 92% precision on car 'slide' prediction), confirming the validation step presented above. However, we notice that the trained models show difficulties with exploratory activities (i.e., car 'overturn' and ball 'shake' have a very low recall). Since the quantity and variety of child activity data which is feasible to collect in a real scenario will most likely be not sufficient for a traditional model training, we envision the possibility to apply *transfer learning* methodologies for the classification purposes in our future works.

6   Conclusion

In this paper we exploit current SoA activity recognition methodologies for wearable sensors, applying them on non-worn, non intrusive sensors. More specifically, the mentioned methodologies are applied on a smart toy set developed in the context of the AutoPlay project. We present activity prediction methodologies, trained over in-lab collected data, and capable to predict infant play activity from inertial data collected by sensor nodes embedded within the toys. The usage of non intrusive measurement methodology is beneficial in preserving the infant behaviour while playing, thus in gathering meaningful, reliable and objective data. This aspect is particularly important when the measurement is exploited for clinical observation purposes. Being able to make prediction on acquired data from non-worn, non-intrusive sensors is thus essential. In this paper we have produced an in-lab dataset using the AutoPlay toys, we annotated the activities with the aid of cameras and we trained activity prediction models for a limited set of three toys and four activities per each toy (identified as the most relevant infant activities). The results obtained are really promising: the achieved test accuracy on in-lab data ranges from 71% (for car and elephant toys) to 96% (for a ball toy). Therefore the proposed study demonstrates that the activity recognition applied to sensors data coming from toys embedded sensor nodes has great potentials and that the available technology is ready for such implementation.

Acknowledgements. We would like to acknowledge first of all Emmanuelle Rossini for the definition of the idea at the base of the AutoPlay approach. We acknowledge Dr. Gian Paolo Ramelli and his neuropediatric team of the EOC Hospital in Bellinzona for supporting us in the real use case scenario data collection. We acknowledge Franesca Faraci, Alessandro Puiatti, all the SUPSI DTI and DEASS collaborators of the Auto-Play team which contributed to the collection of the real use case scenarios data, Pepe Hiller and Hape Toys for the AutoPlay toys design and production. Last but not least, we would like to thank all the families and children which trust our project and which agreed to collaborate with us.

References

1. Anguita, D., Ghio, A., Oneto, L., Parra Perez, X., Reyes Ortiz, J.L.: A public domain dataset for human activity recognition using smartphones. In: Proceedings of the 21th International European Symposium on Artificial Neural Networks, Computational Intelligence and Machine Learning, pp. 437–442 (2013)
2. Antar, A.D., Ahmed, M., Ahad, M.A.R.: Challenges in sensor-based human activity recognition and a comparative analysis of benchmark datasets: a review. In: 2019 Joint 8th International Conference on Informatics, Electronics & Vision (ICIEV) and 2019 3rd International Conference on Imaging, Vision and Pattern Recognition (icIVPR), pp. 134–139. IEEE (2019)
3. Bahad, P., Saxena, P.: Study of adaboost and gradient boosting algorithms for predictive analytics. In: Singh Tomar, G., Chaudhari, N.S., Barbosa, J.L.V., Aghwariya M.K. (eds.) International Conference on Intelligent Computing and Smart Communication 2019. Algorithms for Intelligent Systems. Springer, Singapore (2020). https://doi.org/10.1007/978-981-15-0633-8_22
4. Faraci, F.D., et al.: Autoplay: a smart toys-kit for an objective analysis of children ludic behavior and development. In: 2018 IEEE International Symposium on Medical Measurements and Applications (MeMeA), pp. 1–6. IEEE (2018)
5. Mehmood, A., Raza, A., Nadeem, A., Saeed, U.: Study of multi-classification of advanced daily life activities on shimmer sensor dataset. Int. J. Commun. Networks Inf. Secur. **8**(2), 86 (2016)
6. Papandrea, M., Giordano, S.: Location prediction and mobility modelling for enhanced localization solution. J. Ambient. Intell. Humaniz. Comput. **5**(3), 279–295 (2014)
7. Rivera, D., García, A., Alarcos, B., Velasco, J.R., Ortega, J.E., Martínez-Yelmo, I.: Smart toys designed for detecting developmental delays. Sensors **16**(11), 1953 (2016)
8. Sguazza, S., et al.: Sensor data synchronization in a IoT environment for infants motricity measurement. In: EAI International Conference on IoT Technologies for HealthCare, pp. 3–21. Springer, Cham (2019). https://doi.org/10.1007/978-3-030-42029-1_1

9. Shimmer: Shimmer faqs. http://www.shimmersensing.com/support/wireless-sensor-networks-faqs/
10. Svetnik, V., Liaw, A., Tong, C., Culberson, J.C., Sheridan, R.P., Feuston, B.P.: Random forest: a classification and regression tool for compound classification and QSAR modeling. J. Chem. Inf. Comput. Sci. **43**(6), 1947–1958 (2003)
11. Westeyn, T.L., Abowd, G.D., Starner, T.E., Johnson, J.M., Presti, P.W., Weaver, K.A.: Monitoring children's developmental progress using augmented toys and activity recognition. Pers. Ubiquit. Comput. **16**(2), 169–191 (2012)

Human-Centered Computing - Ubiquitous and Mobile Computing

Co-design the Acceptability of Wearables in the Healthcare Field

Paolo Perego$^{(\boxtimes)}$ ⓘ, Martina Scagnoli ⓘ, and Roberto Sironi

Design Department, Politecnico di Milano, Milan, Italy
{paolo.perego,martina.scagnoli,roberto.sironi}@polimi.it

Abstract. Nowadays, health is perceived as autonomy, both in the management and assessment of care processes. With Wearable Technology, tech companies and national health services move healthcare in everyday life to a better life. Wearables are already functionally high performing, but they still have acceptability and usability issues, especially in digital immigrants. Mobile health could contribute to patient empowerment in the digital health revolution if the human feels fulfilled by the new experience proposed.

This paper presents a case study of co-design and co-evaluation applied to a wearable service system for monitoring and driving self-rehabilitation at home. The participatory approach has been used to investigate the complex relationship between technical and human factors. Rapid Prototyping allows for developing tangible tools as testing and communication one. The different users and stakeholders involved in the project used the prototypes as tangible interfaces to understand and share their needs. The goal of this iterative process of interaction and reflection is to design a quality user experience.

This paper aims to show how design-driven methods and tools can effectively conduct Research-through-Design to increase the acceptability of wearable systems. The positive results of the usability tests during the Multimodal Wearable case study show that wearable systems' acceptability depends on the perceived user-friendliness, which is strictly connected to the co-design process.

Keywords: Wearable · HCI · Research-through-Design (RtD) · Co-design

1 Introduction

Developments in Information Technology (IT) led to an improvement in people's quality of life. The Internet of Things (IoT) remodels the Healthcare system, making it ubiquitous and increasingly a home centered [1] and person-centered care. It has been recognized that the domestic context, with its familiar atmosphere [2], offers a better and faster healing experience and quality of care. It has been demonstrated, especially during the global COVID 19 pandemic when

S. Spinsante et al. (Eds.): HealthyIoT 2021, LNICST 432, pp. 21–32, 2022.
https://doi.org/10.1007/978-3-030-99197-5_2

people have learned to reset much of their lives within their home and proximity spaces, that connected digital devices are a potential medium to interact with the outside world. Personal Health Systems (PHSs) are playing an essential role in providing an at-home system of cure, monitoring, prevention, and a personalised care, since are developed and tailored with the patient for better treatment [3,4].

In the last years, electronic and mechanical miniaturization brought compact computing devices into clothing and other accessories that can be worn comfortably on the body [5]. A wearable device is usually an intelligent object which can include sensors, actuators, smart fabrics, power supplies, Wireless Communication Networks (WCNs), processing units, and multimedia devices [6]. Wearables can be used in various end-user lifestyle sectors, offering the same possibility to receive continuous personal monitoring and access information anytime and anywhere [7].

In the medical sector, Smart Wearable Devices (SWDs) have been diffused from the late 1990s as Wearable Health Devices (WHDs) to help in "patient empowerment" [8]. Smart wearable technologies, with sensory and scanning features such as biofeedback and tracking of physiological function, enable remote monitoring healthcare services to help manage patients' health and well-being [6]. Although wearables are mature from a technological point of view, it has been noted that the adoption and diffusion of these in medical eld are relatively low [7]. Most wearables have a short life cycle, and user acceptance in medicine is still not as widespread as expected [9]. As part of PHS technologies, despite the advantages they offer to various health and social care systems [4], they seem to have not yet had a rapid spread.

Wearables are not yet fully accepted because often understanding how they work is not easy, the way they are used does not feel natural, and therefore the potential that wearables have to offer is not even understood. For example, research on adopting SWDs to assist healthcare in China examined the potential factors affecting user adoption. The study found that the influence of trust on users' attitudes towards SWDs was the most significant, which is followed by compatibility, perceived usefulness (PU), and perceived ease of use (PEOU) [6].

How to solve the problems of acceptability and usability of wearables? By considering human needs and competences that are strongly linked to the type of users (digital natives or digital migrants) within the design and development methodology. Human Centered Design (HCD) tools help to analyze the real contexts of use for which to design, and participatory design tools help to co-design with the real users of those same contexts, including them for all intents and purposes in the design team made up of all project stakeholders. Since wearables are service hubs that can act as active or passive interfaces [10], it is essential to have a broader system view and focus on the design of relations and interactions complexity about technology-to-person services. This challenge requires a multi-stakeholder process of Product Service System (PSS) design [4] conducted with a design-driven approach. This paper shows the development method used during a co-design and co-evaluation case study for remotely monitored rehabilitation wearable service systems. The method has implemented a participatory approach with various stakeholders and users to improve usability and acceptability, investigating and testing the relationships between technical and human factors in developing the wearable system.

2 Reflecting on the Contribution of Design to Enhance the Wearables' Acceptability

The IoT has enabled digital PSSs to capture and exchange data, creating a network of ubiquitously connected devices within our physical and social spaces. Nowadays, technology permeates most aspects of everyone's life: smartphones have become the most indispensable personal mobile tool to interact with, allowing to act passively and actively on the world. Wearables then are more complex devices and require hybrid designs. They come from the synergy between multiple science domains - such as biomedical technologies, micro, and nanotechnologies, materials engineering, electronic engineering, and information and communication technologies [12].

HCD methodologies and holistic design requirements identification tools, help build an overview of technical and human factors [13], from different stakeholder perspectives, which can be used as a canvas to visualize and draw potential relationships to be implemented in the project. This article aims to show the contribution of the phenomenological design approach to improve the acceptability of wearables. In particular, we consider the double diamond model to describe the process of acquiring and defining design requirements, focusing on its valid iterative progression and the possibility of creating several research/analysis/test/evaluation loops simultaneously. Designing acceptability means focusing on UX design by analyzing user attitudes and intentions in adopting the proposed new information system from time to time [6]. Early acceptability design concept translates into the involvement of the different users and stakeholders, from the earliest stages of the production process. Since the user acceptance of wearables depends on transversal socio-technical relations, and the final usability and satisfaction depend on a combined focus on technical and human challenges, a co-design approach enhances the coexistence of different considerations in the design projects. It encourages dialogue between various experts (including final users). As is the case in Human-Computer Interaction (HCI) studies, it might be helpful to consider each requirement as a combination of both factors (technical and human) and categorize it according to physical, cognitive, and emotional ergonomics [9]. Additionally, verification and validation are necessary to define them according to their specific evaluation technique and the degree of development at which the process is [9]. Prototyping is a promising tool to support the different definition phases of the digital PSS development, the co-design process, and knowledge sharing techniques about intangible elements by fostering an iterative and interactive process of co-evaluation [11].

2.1   An Empirical Case Study to Design an Acceptable Wearable PSS

This paper focuses on testing the above-mentioned theoretical concepts, executing, and analyzing a design project for the healthcare sector.

The project, called Multimodal Wearable (MW), was funded by "Centro Protesi" INAIL, one of the research centers of the National Institute for Insurance against Accidents at Work. It aimed to design a wearable system for monitoring and evaluating motor rehabilitation activities in post-stroke patients, offering a more personal and personalized at-home service to conduct Rehabilitation in autonomy. All this conveys the benefits of extending care in the home environment to improve the quality of the rehabilitation experience during the recovery period, accelerate the healing process of the injured worker, and speed up his or her reintegration into work [15]. For the different contexts that the project would touch, designing with a horizontal and holistic vision was mandatory to make it arise from their intersection. Increasing the performance expected from the new system led to adding some degrees of complexity, causing a potential decrease in usability.

The Octopus methodology [14] was used as the primary reference to organize the different human-centered design principles provided by ISO 9241 and the different collaborative design-evaluation and review phases the MW project and its stakeholders provided. The iterative nature of the Octopus methodology has helped the project better define itself in its complexity, expanding the methodology [15] toward the design of the User Experience (UX) and the User Interaction (UI) of the Internet of the body.

To design for the new scenario of use resulting from the intersection of the rehabilitation and domestic contexts and the human body as a surface for wearables, the following were explored in-depth:

- User Experience and the network of interactions between users and the wearables' system.
- Wearability and human factors.

Approaching human performance from a data perspective could mean relying on quantitative, objectively valid sources to focus on the design of qualitatively more appropriate and effective communication. The new technology and interactive experience emerged from the systematization of information from desk and shared context analyses. Interviews, focus groups, and participatory design actions have supported the design team and the MW project stakeholders to conduct the User Research in the real context.

In the rehabilitation center, chosen as a reference environment, two focus groups were led, and ad-hoc questionnaires were administered to 30 participants [15].

Through the questionnaire, during the first focus group, the design team wanted to investigate the response of patients and technologists on different issues such as preferences in the detection of wearable system parameters, wearability, morphology and modularity of the wearable system, aspects related to the interface and user/system interaction and engagement levels, elements about usability and aesthetic acceptability. There were two types of users: the patient, as a wearer, and primary/direct user of the wearable or also called Actor User (AU), and the technologist as a secondary user and part of the Professional Users (PU), who can process the collected data and indirectly guide and monitor the patient parameters [14]. Both patients and technologists are interested in monitoring biomechanical data and those more related to movement. For both, the wearable system needs to motivate and follow the patient in the rehabilitation path through a dedicated interface (APP or other). Consequently, patients prefer to interface with the wearable system through the smartphone. The PUs supports the importance of having real-time data to monitor and evaluate the rehabilitation activity or having data available at the end of the session. Patients would like to send the data immediately after the training is completed. In general, according to the patient's pathology, they agree to opt for a wearable system divided by body districts, who prefer to receive a complete configured system from the PUs. For PUs, the comfort aspect of the wearable is an essential aspect to consider, compared to AUs, who assume that wearing time aspects are more relevant. The workshop has been used to have either an aesthetically discreet and almost invisible system concept or a customizable one to manage the aesthetic level independently.

Through these participatory design tools, it is shown how users were considered active members from the beginning of the MW project. Therefore, the different stakeholders involved in the co-design team were:

- Patients with different pathologies from the rehabilitation center.
- Physicians, technologists, and healthcare workers from the rehabilitation center.
- Technologists from INAIL.
- Technologists and Designers from the design team.

This first co-design session highlighted human and technical factors from different user perspectives. The first level of contextual factors defined the choice of technologies to be implemented and the preferred modes of interaction. The technological study then took three parallel development paths towards the setting of:

- A Wearable system.
- A smart garment.
- An APP for smartphone.

The APP has the double task as Data visualization and Data Processing Point (DPP) [14]. The second focus group has been administered with patients and therapists to deepen the requirements related to preferences about usability, Graphical User Interface (GUI), wearable aesthetic, time and space of use. The patients involved in the focus groups and survey were working-age people following a hospitalized rehabilitation path due to myoplasia or post-stroke. Thanks to this double patient type, focus groups have the further objective of assessing

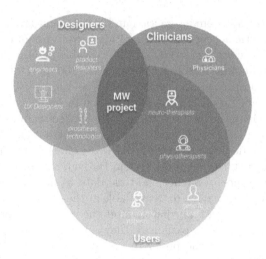

Fig. 1. Representation of MW Project's stakeholder.

how the same aspects were received and characterized according to the type of pathology. Another mandatory evaluation has been related to data visualization and storing. Through interviews, it has also been possible to understand which data to display, how, where, and how to store/process/send them. In general, operators required a simple management system focused on physical and cognitive ergonomics. Patients need the simplicity of use, ease of wearing, cleanliness, breathability, and therefore parameters linked to the effectiveness and usability of the system, rather than aesthetics. The comment: "I would like it to look like an everyday object", was very explanatory. To complete identifying user-side requirements in the domestic context, a questionnaire has been administered to new users to be filled in online. In this questionnaire, the user had to reply about the relationship between their fitness status, physical activities practiced in the domestic context, and the possible presence of musculoskeletal pathologies where relevant. The participants had to assess some parameters based on the indices of time spent, posture taken, body district affected, and the level of perceived fatigue. In the final part, questions related to the user's work activity were also proposed to assess the user's attitude to use wearables for risk prevention at work. The results have shown that, for the interviewed, the most exciting aspects of being monitored are the feedback about postures during home and work activities and the stress related to these. This collaboration process during analysis, synthesis, sharing, and reflection with the project's various users and stakeholders led to a balancing of the design requirements according to physical, cognitive, and the users' experience (e.g., from direct use to the emotional aspects). Thanks to the iterative process, typical of user centered design approach, co-design could be led since the beginning of the design process.

2.2   Improve Wearable Acceptability Through UX and UI Design

After the first analysis with focus groups, interviews, and questionnaires, quantitative and qualitative data have been gathered to apply the so-called mixed method for collecting "what and why", related to acceptability and usability problems. Defining a good interaction with wearable devices means integrating data evaluated in the previous phase to design the most appropriate, intuitive, and uncomplicated experience for users. The content and representation of the information to be shared must be adequate to each mental profile that should receive it and to the context of reception [14]. How can the patient better understand and interact with all the wearable system components and proactively improve his/her healthcare service? How to create a transparent system architecture and design simple patient actions?

The Multimodal Wearable project has been chosen to resolve system complexity by designing a smart garment with fixed wearable marks. This led to the definition of a modular multi-parameter wearable system, available in upper, lower, or upper/lower versions. The positions of the inertial modules for sensing biomechanical data and the module for monitoring physiological data depended on the body districts to be monitored. The decision to create garments with the wearable system receptacles already in place was driven by the desire to help users by providing them with a near-complete solution that was easy to wear and use autonomously, by placing the right wearables in the proper receptacle. The positioning of wearable has been designed focusing on the guidance of affordance. For Norman, affordance is an object's design aspect that suggests how the object should be used, a visual clue to its function and use. Affordance refers to the perceived and actual properties of the thing [16]. The existence of an affordance depends upon the properties of both the product and the user's perception. The design team mapped out areas of the body where wearables would be less invasive and, at the same time, more effective for sensing biomechanical body movements and physiological parameters. Design for wearability and comfort also consider aesthetic and social acceptability values in the definition of proper body areas [17]. Creating shapes that recall everyday objects helps people contact technology and increase acceptability and usability. For this reason, the device has a shape inspired by polished stones used for relaxing massages. Simple experience indicates that compact short shapes, like those of stones or control knobs, invite to be contacted by a fingertip grip [16]. Moreover, to ensure the uniqueness of positioning and coupling between the wearable and the receptacle positioned on the smart garment, and not to generate frustration during the wearability phase, were considered:

- Positioning strategy.
- Shape orientation.
- Docking system to the garment.
    - to co-reflect with other project users and stakeholders and improve from a usability perspective.
    - fixing system
- Charging case.

To address the correct wearable positioning on the smart garment, the strategy of making same-colored markers for each device/position pair was adopted. Considerations about wearable shape orientation on the on the garment, conduct the design team to pursue two roads at the same time:

- The definition of an asymmetrical top/bottom shape (to ensure the correct electrical contact).
- Same outline for wearable and receptacle to maximize contact stiffness.

A magnetic coupling/contact type capable of ensuring mechanical and electrical tightness and comfort during the coupling process was developed from a technological perspective. While implementing different design requirements, the design team first used various CAD/CAE tools and inspirational mock-ups to co-design affordance. Therefore, rapid prototyping has allowed to materialize them to test their effectiveness with the final user in a real-life context.

Using a range of production techniques and technologies, both additive and traditional, it was possible to harmoniously combine hard and soft parts in the same object to maximize wearability and comfort. It was possible to use different 3D printing materials to obtain simple conceptual models and functional multi-material prototypes to study and understand the interaction. At the same time, the relationship between the size of the wearable device (depending mainly on the implemented technology and battery) and its position on the body was achieved concerning human factors considerations. The communication and networking part of the system, also related to user-product interaction, was iteratively designed, prototyped, and co-evaluated through users' tests. MW wearables showed system state and error by a multi-color LED included in the input button [15]; this aspect about error and feedback has also been discussed with users who prefer, as Norman indicates [18], to be aware of the system's status. From this point of view, Smartphone APP was another important part of the feedback. The APP has been thought not only to display collected data but also to help the user during system configuration, let him aware of it in case of error, device problem, or battery consumption. Users participated in making the GUI design more understandable by testing its application of Nielsen's heuristics [18]. Real tests were possible since the same smartphone could connect to multiple devices via Bluetooth. Users could test the proposed MW experience with an actual high-fidelity prototype shown in Fig. 1.

The last co-design session was mainly in a Rehabilitation center (Ospedale Riabilitativo Valduce Villa Beretta" di Costa Masnaga). A panel of ten healthy subjects tested four complete MW systems (smart garment, wearables, and APP). Test on subjects with pathologies was not conducted for safety reasons due to the actual Covid 19 pandemic; they evaluated the system without wearing it. The high-fidelity MW prototypes were assessed according to the parameters of:

- The kinematic accuracy of the biomechanical model of the shoulder district, according to a validation protocol developed by the Rehabilitation center.
- The usability test (evaluation of ergonomics and aesthetic acceptability) using an ad hoc developed SUS (System Usability Scale) questionnaire (Fig. 2).

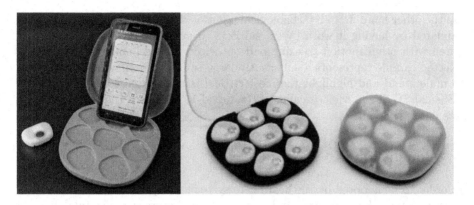

Fig. 2. Prototypes of the hard components and the GUI of the MW system.

Healthy subjects and therapists performed wearability tests and biometric surveys. Subsequently, they were administered to a standardized questionnaire (SUS - System Usability Scale) [19]. and other questions based on the Likert scale to measure the degree of acceptability of the system. The results of this evaluation showed an excellent adherence between the high initial expectations of the subjects involved and the post-test evaluation of the system. This means that the system has responded to the expected needs of the users.

In general, the perceived quality of the system was high, and this value was substantially confirmed by the totality of the parameters analyzed in the usability assessment. It should be emphasized that the system's quality of the information received, the overall acceptance, and the appropriateness of the operations carried out by MW reached an optimal score (¿6/7). At the same time, the other evaluation parameters were at very good values, close to the optimal; slightly lower the scores related to wearability (4.1/5) and aesthetic acceptability (5.40/7). In particular, the values of these two parameters underline the opportunity to improve the system by intervening on suit aesthetics and dressing and undressing method. The usability test also measured the wearing times of the system, which was around 4 min for dressing and around 1 min and 30 s for undressing, which are acceptable values when compared with normal clothes dressing. Results showed excellent adherence between the high initial expectations of the project's stakeholders and the post-test evaluation of the MW system. The quality of the information received by the system, the overall acceptance, and the appropriateness of the operations carried out by MW achieved an optimum score. At the same time, the other evaluation parameters have been significant. Wearability and aesthetic acceptability have been rated good. Users asked for improvements to the opening system in the smart garment (to facilitate especially wearability by patients with hemiparesis) and increase sizing. The system application obtained, in general, a good evaluation, SUS score 75.5/100, which becomes optimal when looking at the therapists' data 87.5/100. This demonstrates the effectiveness of the new methodologies adopted [15].

On the other hand, from a technological point of view, the MW system has been validated by having it worn by six subjects to perform the function test compared with other motion tracking and optoelectronic technology systems. The selected sample represents a sufficiently large sample of users and stakeholders to understand and highlight the most critical issues related to the usability of PSSs [20, 21] due to the criticality of the Covid-19 breakout, the sample of users was not expanded.

3   Conclusion

In order to be adopted by the healthcare system, in a pervasive healthcare perspective, and to be recognized and accepted by end-users as understandable and practical, wearable should be developed with the user at the center of the design process, and by taking co-design approach as the right one to deal with users' needs, acceptance and usability. This increases the completeness of the result expected by those who will be the final users of the project, having started from their needs. It is a matter of defining the starting point well, analyzing it from both human and technical points of view, to create a solution as close as possible to the needs discovered at that point. Adopting human-centered tools help to explore a technological-driven field like Wearable Technology with a design-driven approach, giving more importance to aspects related to the human side of the experience. Maintaining users at the center facilitates the objectives and constraints identification and the design gap definition. Then, discussions between the various stakeholders help to co-evaluate and co-reflect on the multiple outcomes of the prototyping process that functioned as rapid cycles of collaborative learning. Moreover, prototypes played a central role in the process of thinking about how design could influence the improved acceptability of wearables since they allowed:

– To support each design team component to reflect on its ideas.
– To share ideas within the design team.
– To co-reflect on the prototyping process and progress it.
– To test the solutions created in the real context and co-reflect with other project users and stakeholders.

In this way, it is possible to simultaneously assess body-centered issues, material selection, technology, product-user communication, physical ergonomics, and comfort issues from both performance and usability points of view. This approach has been tested during the development of the Multimodal Wearable system for motor rehabilitation, obtaining good results in terms of design outcome for users' expectations and needs. The test analysis has shown that the system has good approval ratings from most of the rehabilitation process actors: users, caregivers, and clinicians.

Acknowledgments. This work has been supported by "Centro Protesi INAIL" - Vigorso di Budrio (BO), Italy, the main research center of the National Institute for

Insurance against Accidents at Work. The authors would also like to thank all the focus group participants for their willingness and patience, and to eng. Angelo Davalli, eng Emanuele Gruppioni and eng. Rinaldo Sacchetti of INAIL Centro Protesi for supervising the research.

References

1. Rahmani, A.M., et al.: Smart e-Health gateway: bringing intelligence to Internet-of-Things based ubiquitous healthcare systems. In: 12th Annual IEEE Consumer Communications and Networking Conference. CCNC 2015, pp. 826–834 (2015)
2. Lupton, D.: The digitally engaged patient: self-monitoring and self-care in the digital health era. Soc. Theory Heal. **11**(3), 256–270 (2013)
3. Flores, M., Glusman, G., Brogaard, K., Price, N.D., Hood, L.: P4 medicine: how systems medicine will transform the healthcare sector and society. Per. Med. **10**(6), 565–576 (2013)
4. Schartinger, D., et al.: Technology Innovation Management Review Personal Health Systems Technologies: Critical Issues in Service Innovation and Diffusion (2015)
5. Wright, R., Keith, L.: Wearable technology: if the tech fits, wear it. J. Electron. Resour. Med. Libr. **11**(4), 204–216 (2014)
6. Gao, S., Zhang, X., Peng, S.: Understanding the adoption of smart wearable devices to assist healthcare in China. In: Social Media: The Good, the Bad, and the Ugly, pp. 280–291 (2016)
7. Niknejad, N., Ismail, W.B., Mardani, A., Liao, H., Ghani, H.: A comprehensive overview of smart wearables: the state of the art literature, recent advances, and future challenges. Eng. Appl. Artif. Intell. **90**, 103529 (2020)
8. Dias, D., Cunha, J.P.S.: Wearable health devices-vital sign monitoring, systems and technologies. Sensors (Switzerland) **18**(8) (2018). (MDPI AG)
9. Francés-Morcillo, L., Morer-Camo, P., Rodríguez-Ferradas, M.I., Cazón-Martín, A.: Wearable design requirements identification and evaluation. Sensors (Switzerland) **20**(9) (2020)
10. Francés-Morcillo, L., Morer-Camo, P., Rodríguez-Ferradas, M.I., Cazón-Martín, A.: The role of user-centred design in smart wearable systems design process. Proc. Int. Des. Conf. Des. **5**(1), 2197–2208 (2018)
11. Kleinsmann, M., Ten Bhömer, M.: The (New) roles of prototypes during the co-development of digital product service systems. Int. J. Des. **14**(1), 65–79 (2020)
12. Dias, D., Cunha, J.P.S.: Wearable health devices-vital sign monitoring, systems and technologies. Sensors (Switzerland) **18**(8) (2018)
13. Morcillo, L.F., Morer-Camo, P., Ferradas, M.I.R., Martín, A.C.: The wearable co-design domino: a user-centered methodology to co-design and co-evaluate wearables. Sensors (Switzerland) **20**(10) (2020)
14. Marin, J., Blanco, T., Marin, J.J.: Octopus: a design methodology for motion capture wearables. Sensors (Switzerland) **17**(8), 1–24 (2017)
15. Perego, P., Sironi, R., Scagnoli, M., Fusca, M., Gruppioni, E., Davalli, A.: Multimodal Wearable System for Motor Rehabilitation - Design Perspective and Development, pp. 99–106 (2021)
16. Wolf, A., Krüger, D., Miehling, J., Wartzack, S.: Approaching an ergonomic future: an affordance-based interaction concept for digital human models. Procedia CIRP **84**, 520–525 (2019)
17. Zeagler, C., Gandy, M., Baker, P.: The assistive wearable: inclusive by design. Assist. Technol. Outcomes Benefits (ATOB) **12** (2018)

18. Nielsen, J.: Ten usability heuristics (2005)
19. Kortum, P.T., Bangor, A.: Usability ratings for everyday products measured with the system usability scale. Int. J. Hum. Comput. Interact. **29**(2), 67–76 (2013)
20. Lewis, J.R.: Sample sizes for usability studies: additional considerations. Hum. Factors **36**, 368–378 (1994)
21. Nielsen, J., Landauer, T.K.: A mathematical model of the finding of usability problems. In: Proceedings of the INTERACT'93 and CHI'93 Conference on Human Factors in Computing Systems, pp. 206–213 (1993)

Evaluations on Pending Regulation on Ethical Review Measures for Biomedical Research Involving Human Subjects and Artificial Intelligence

Xiaoyu Sun[✉]

Beijing National Day School, Beijing, China
wuan0423@qq.com

Abstract. The rapid development of Artificial Intelligence (AI) has extensively promoted medicine, pharmaceutical, and other related fields in recent years. The ethics review is one of the critical procedures of registration to get the medical artificial intelligence products approved and commercialized. The National Health Commission of the People's Republic of China published a consultation paper on the Ethical Review Measures for Biomedical Research Involving Human Beings (Second Version) (the Draft) on March 16th, 2021.

Although the Draft indicated that the Ethics Review Committees need to be set up by the Regional and Institutional level, the review authorities of different levels were not clarified. The suggestion is that three tiers of Ethics Review Committees should be set up in China. The precise scope of review authorities for each level should be identified. Such as the complicated leading technology, gene editing, should be reviewed by National Ethics Review Committees. It will be the job of individual institute Ethics Review Committees to approve the clinical research with less risk such as a new ointment to treat acne. Furthermore, to standardize the research and development of artificial intelligence in healthcare in the age of AI, more clear guidance should be given to data security in the layers of data, algorithm, and application in the ethics review process. In addition, transparency and responsibility, as two of six principles in the Rome Call for AI Ethics promoted by the Pontifical Academy for Life and presented on February 28th, 2020, could be further strengthened in the Draft.

Keywords: Biomedical research involving human beings · Data security · Ethics Committees · Ethical Review · Medical artificial intelligence

1 Introduction

The rapid development of Artificial Intelligence (AI) has extensively promoted medicine, pharmaceutical, and other related fields in recent years. There is an expectation that the implications of AI can have a significant positive impact on quality of care of patients, disease prevention, diagnosis, and treatment options, in addition to the potential for

S. Spinsante et al. (Eds.): HealthyIoT 2021, LNICST 432, pp. 33–38, 2022.
https://doi.org/10.1007/978-3-030-99197-5_3

efficiency gains and reduction in human error. The research and development of artificial intelligence in healthcare by scientific and commercial organizations are on the fast track. The ethics review is one of the critical procedures of registration to get the products quickly approved and launched.

However, the Standard Operating Procedures for ethics review is not enough to guide the healthy and rapid development of artificial intelligence in healthcare in China. Ethical Review Measures for Biomedical Research Involving Human Beings were enacted by the National Health Commission of the People's Republic of China (NHC) on December 1st, 2016 [1]. However, from a legislative design perspective, it was neither updated timely nor in line with the international trends of AI development. Therefore, it was great that NHC published a consultation paper on the Ethical Review Measures for Biomedical Research Involving Human Beings (Second Version) (the Draft) on March 16th, 2021 [2], and started to collect public comments on the Draft.

2 Methods

In order to submit the comments to the Draft and facilitate AI development in China, first, the laws and regulations in the USA and EU were reviewed and compared, then 11 subject matter experts (SMEs) in China were in-depth interviewed (IDI), including lawmakers, regulators, and key members of ethics review committees, heads of Regulatory Affairs in Software as a Medical Device (SaMD) industry, and data scientists. The tailor-made questionnaire for each SME was prepared, interviewed each SME in 75 min from April to June. Coupled with the findings from the global laws and regulations, the opinions of SMEs were summarized and enlighten on the proposed suggestions to the Draft [2].

3 Results and Discussion

3.1 Ethics Review Committees in Three Tiers (Institutional, Provincial, and National) Should Be Established in China While Identifying the Clear, Precise Scope of Review Authorities for Each Level

The Draft indicated that the Institutional Review Board (IRB) and Regional Ethics Committee (REC) need to be set up for ethics review. The responsibility of IRB was specified as IRB provides an ethical review of human subjects research to be conducted in the institution or delegated institution, to protect the rights and welfare of human subjects of research and to assure that human research is conducted according to applicable national, provincial, and local laws and regulations and the relevant policies. However, the responsibility of REC was not indicated in the Draft, and the review authorities of IRB and REC were not clarified.

Chinese Hospital Association and the Ethics Expert Committee of NHC released the Guidance to Ethics Review Committee for Clinical Research Involving Human Beings in October 2020, but no guidance for the limits of authorities of IRB and REC [3].

The United States of American and European countries set up REC much earlier, the experiences of those countries could be referred to improve and perfect the regulations in China:

The United States of American. Several RECs were established in the USA. For example, the Biomedical Research Alliance of New York (BRANY) was founded in 1998 by four nationally-ranked academic medical centers. BRANY IRB was the first IRB in New York to be accredited by Association for the Accreditation of Human Research Protection Program (AAHRPP) in 2006, takes the role of REC to oversee the researches involving human subjects in the region [4, 5].

Western Institutional Review Board (WIRB) is an independent central IRB located in Puyallup, Washington, oversights overall human participant research at Wayne State University (WSU) and its affiliates registered under the Wayne State Federal wide Assurance (FWA). WIRB also takes the role of REC, cooperated with more than 100 research centers and pharmaceutical companies to review their research projects in the region [4, 6].

The United Kingdom. The United Kingdom Ethics Committees Authority (UKECA) was founded in 2004 to authorize and oversee the operation of IRBs in the UK; UKECA identifies IRBs by three types. The type II IRB takes the responsibilities of REC to review and approve the researches in its region [4, 7].

Sweden. Six RECs were established by geographical location [8]. Therefore, the principal investigator (PI) of a multiple center clinical trial should get approval from one REC where PI's institution locates in. Then the approval is effective national wide.

Those countries have the practice of RECs. However, no specific guidance is developed to link the risk levels of the research with the review authorities of ethics committees at each level.

In the age of AI, biomedical research projects have become more complex, the potential risks are more difficult to be forecasted. To be more efficient, biomedical researches with risks at different levels should be reviewed and approved by ethics committees at a different levels. Three tiers of ethics review committees should be established in China. They are Institutional Review Board (IRB), Provincial Ethics Committee (PEC), and National Ethics Committee (NEC). For example, the clinical research of a new ointment to treat acne has less risks, IRB could review and approve it independently. The risks of some research are not high, but unique populations such as psychiatric patients are involved, or about certain diseases such as rare diseases or organ transplantations, IRB should review first and then submit to PEC for approval. The complicated leading technology, such as Assisted Reproductive Technology (ART), Gene editing, Mitochondrial Replacement Techniques (MRT), Interspecies Cloning, etc., have high risks, should be preliminary reviewed by IRB, second reviewed by REC, finally approved by NEC (Table 1).

3.2 The Guidance About Data Security in Ethics Review Should Be Clearly Described in the Draft

The Draft has minimal guidance to IRB in data security, majorly focuses on data sharing and secondary utilization. In the age of AI, more AI will be involved in biomedical research, such as Software as a Medical Device (SaMD), data security has been an essential topic. Strengthening data security and privacy protection is the key to researching,

Table 1. The Scope of Review Authorities of the Ethics Committees in Different Level

Risk levels	IRB	REC	NEC
Researches with low or medium risks	Approval		
Researches with low or medium risks: Special population: psychiatric patients etc Special diseases: rare diseases, organ transplantations etc	Review	Approval	
Researches with high risks [9]: Assisted Reproductive Technology (ART), Gene Editing, Mitochondrial Replacement Techniques (MRT), Interspecies cloning, etc.	Preliminary review	Second review	Approval

developing, and applying medical artificial intelligence. The USA and some European countries have adopted policies for critical privacy data related to medical, such as increasing the difficulty of cracking by strong encryption and establishing strict data access procedures and authorities [10].

The research of medical artificial intelligence products is inseparable from patients' health data and medical record data. Therefore, the Draft should give more explicit guidance to ethics review in data security in the kind research. The Draft should identify the ethics review requirement for data security and privacy protection, including the qualification of the research personnel who may have direct contact with the research data, infrastructure, access control technologies, etc., to ensure data security and privacy protection in the data layer, algorithm layer, and application layer in the entire research process [11].

3.3 Transparency and Responsibility Should Be Supplemented into the Principles of Ethics Review

The Draft identified eight principles of ethics review in biomedical research. They were Compliance, Informed Consent, Control Risk, Fairness, Free and Compensation, Privacy Protection, Special Protection, and Public Interests [2].

Transparency and responsibility were the principles in almost all the regulations and guidelines related to AI Ethics in the USA and European countries [12]. The "Rome Call for AI Ethics" promoted the use of Artificial Intelligence-based on Transparency, Inclusion, Responsibility, Impartiality, Reliability, Security, and Privacy principles [13]. The Call, promoted by the Pontifical Academy for Life and presented on February 28, 2020, had as first signatories the President of Microsoft Brad Smith, the Vice President of IBM John Kelly III, the Director-General of the Food and Agriculture Organization of the United Nations (FAO) Qu Dongju and the Minister for Innovation of the Italian Government Paola Pisano.

Transparency. To realize the principle of transparency depends on the explicability, verifiability, and predictability of algorithms of medical artificial intelligence products

[14]. Therefore, when the biomedical research related to medical artificial intelligence is reviewed, the Ethics Committees should ensure that healthcare professionals know how and why medical artificial intelligence makes specific decisions in the research protocol design.

Responsibility. The principle of responsibility means that the Ethics Committees should review if a transparent responsibility system has been established for technology research and development, in order to ensure the technology researchers and design departments can be held accountable from the technical level when medical artificial intelligence product leads to the conflict of human ethics or law [14].

The ethical review of the research related to medical artificial intelligence products has the universality with AI, transparency and responsibility are critical principles of AI ethics, so both should be supplemented into the principles of the Draft.

4 Conclusions

To facilitate the rapid and healthy development of artificial intelligence in healthcare in China, an updated Ethical Review Measures for Biomedical Research Involving Human Beings is essential. On top of the Draft released on March 16th, 2021, suggest establishing Ethics Committees in three tiers with the different authorities. Furthermore, give more explicit guidance on data security in ethics review. In addition, supplement the principles of transparency and responsibility. If the Draft could adopt the suggestions, the efficiency of ethics review will be improved, the human subjects in the biomedical research will be safer, and the process of registration, approval, and commercialization will be expedited. Then China could be one of the most advanced countries in artificial intelligence in healthcare soon.

References

1. The National Health Commission of the People's Republic of China (NHC), The ethical review measures for biomedical research involving human beings, 12th October 2016. http://www.nhc.gov.cn/cms-search/xxgk/getManuscriptXxgk.htm?id=84b33b81d8e7 47eaaf048f68b174f829. Accessed 23 Aug 2021
2. The National Health Commission of the People's Republic of China (NHC), The ethical review measures for biomedical research involving human beings (second version, the Draft), 16th March 2021. http://www.nhc.gov.cn/cms-search/xxgk/getManuscriptXxgk.htm?id=beb 66b1525e64472b1a9b8921ed1aedf. Accessed 23 Aug 2021
3. Chinese Hospital Association and the Ethics Expert Committee of NHC, The guidance to ethics review committee for clinical research involving human beings (v2020), 26th October 2020. http://cctmis.org/zcfg/zc/809.html, Accessed 23 Aug 2021
4. Wang, J.: Development and orientation of regional ethics committee. In: 2018 Annual Conference of Pharmaceutical Clinical Evaluation Research Professional Committee, pp. 45–49. China Pharmaceutical Association (2018)
5. Corporate Overview of BRANY (Biomedical Research Alliance of New York). https://www.brany.com/corporate-overview/. Accessed 23 Aug 2021
6. Introduction of Western Institutional Review Board (WIRB). https://research.wayne.edu/irb/wirb. Accessed 23 Aug 2021

7. Ji, P.: UK research ethics review system introduction and implication. Med. Philos. **41**(9), 30–33 (2020)
8. Wang, Y., He, Y., Luo, X., Ma, X., Zhang, N.: The discussion of ethical review program construction in clinical research. Chinese Med. Ethics **28**(6), 916–918 (2015)
9. The National Health Commission of the People's Republic of China (NHC), Regulation on the administration of clinical application of new biomedical technologies, 26th February 2019. http://www.nhc.gov.cn/wjw/yjzj/201902/0f24ddc242c24212abc42aa8b539584d.shtml. Accessed 23 Aug 2021
10. Xie, X., He, X., Zhang, L., Li, W., Gao, Y.: Analysis on the key points of ethical review concerning medical artificial intelligence research. Chin. Med. Eth. **34**(7), 844–850(2021)
11. Li, L.: Data Ethics and Algorithm Ethics, 1st edn, pp. 83–93. Science Press, Beijing (2019)
12. The National Committee of Artificial Intelligence Standardization, Report to Risk Analysis of AI Ethics, pp. 3–6 (2019). https://pan.baidu.com/s/1uqfLuQB0jEDG0AlDIwWEAA,passcode:c91b. Accessed 23 Aug 2021
13. The Pontifical Academy for Life, Rome Call for AI Ethics. http://www.academyforlife.va/content/pav/en/news/2020/intelligenza-artificiale-2020.html. Accessed 23 Aug 2021
14. The National Committee of Artificial Intelligence Standardization, Report to Risk Analysis of AI Ethics, pp. 31–32 (2019). https://pan.baidu.com/s/1uqfLuQB0jEDG0AlDIwWEAA,passcode:c91b. Accessed 23 Aug 2021

Integration of Wearable, Persuasive, and Multimedia Design Principles in Enhancing Depression Awareness: A Conceptual Model

Umi Hanim Mazlan[1]([⊠]), Siti Mahfuzah Sarif[2], Sobihatun Nur Abdul Salam[2],
Nur Fadziana Faisal Mohamed[2], and Maznah Ibrahim[3]

[1] UiTM Cawangan Perlis, 02600 Arau, Perlis, Malaysia
umihanim462@uitm.edu.my
[2] UUM, 06010 Sintok, Kedah, Malaysia
[3] Ministry of Health Malaysia, KKM, 01000 Kangar, Perlis, Malaysia

Abstract. The prevalence of depression among university students in Malaysia can be reflected in unprecedented suicide acts and attempts among university students across the country. However, there is a scarcity of reliable, practical, and comprehensive methods to curb the issue at the root cause - to empower one's controllability awareness. This study believes that promotion and awareness regarding the pertinent to the importance of mental health problems, especially to specific target groups, can be enhanced through technology. Meanwhile, studies have confirmed the relevance of persuasive methods in wearable technology, though to varying degrees. Persuasive technology has been widely used to create awareness in various domains. Moreover, the multimedia elements could be a value-added property to ensure the effectiveness of the technological solutions in enhancing awareness. Accordingly, this paper discusses constructing a model that integrates wearable, persuasive, and multimedia design principles to enhance one's controllability awareness of depression. The model is constructed through the content analysis method. As a result, a triad of three design principles was consolidated and validated through multidisciplinary expert reviews. This paper discusses the refinement process made to the proposed model, which is aimed to serve as a guideline for developing solutions to enhance controllability awareness on depression issues.

Keywords: Wearable technology · Persuasive technology · Multimedia design · Conceptual model · Controllability awareness · Depression

1 Introduction

The recent National Health and Morbidity Survey reported that 2.3% of adults aged 18 and above in Malaysia experienced depression [1]. According to [2], lack of controllability awareness is the effect of depression and Obsessive-Compulsive Disorder (OCD). Controllability awareness is the ability of an individual to pay attention and differentiate whether the aspects of possible consequences are controllable or uncontrollable in

S. Spinsante et al. (Eds.): HealthyIoT 2021, LNICST 432, pp. 39–49, 2022.
https://doi.org/10.1007/978-3-030-99197-5_4

responding to life situations [3]. Nevertheless, among Malaysian university students, the effects of depression are still unexplored [4] and remain challenging [5]. Accordingly, [6] agreed that it is significant to study the depression problem among students as they have a potential influence on their family, society, and the country and contribute to their country's labour force in the future. Furthermore, as the technology used among mental illness patients is on the rise [7], the promotion and awareness regarding the vitality of mental health problems, especially to specific target groups, can be promoted and enhanced [1] through technology.

1.1 Related Works

Wearable Technology (WT) is a promising means to help individuals develop awareness [8]. In mental health, the capability of WT in capturing behavioural, physiological, and social data related to severe mental illness [9] can be leveraged in enhancing depression awareness among undergraduates. Meanwhile, over the years, persuasive technology also has evolved to deal with diverse practices besides behaviour and attitude [10]. Since the actual transformation in behaviour requires a more extended evaluation period, a review by [10] found that 72% out of 85 studies finally evaluated their system effectiveness by measuring other various outcomes of behaviour-related or psychological including awareness. Moreover, with the help of interactive media, a well-designed application is able to persuade people effectively towards behaviour change [11, 12] as well as influencing them to utilize the technology for learning and sharing information in an interactive way [13].

1.2 Using Content Analysis in Model Development

Content analysis as a research method is an easy-to-use, explicit, and systematic tool for analyzing documents and text, which can be used to develop an understanding and provide new insights and knowledge in different contexts. For instance, [14] applies content analysis for decision criteria, techniques, theories, and Human Computer Interaction (HCI) components to develop a design model for youth personal decision aid. Furthermore, the components and elements in the interactive computer-assisted learning conceptual model were also determined using content analysis [15]. Similarly, [16] conducted content analysis to identify potential solutions from existing solutions for computerized personal-decision aid. Finally, in the study of conceptual design of Reality Learning Media (RLM) model, [17], the content analysis is referred to as the effort to gather basic information at the early stages of study.

Accordingly, this study believes that enhancing controllability awareness can be effective by consolidating all three technologies' design principles. Nevertheless, a previous review of persuasive multimedia principles in wearable technology had confirmed that the absence of the integration of wearable, persuasive and multimedia principles unfold a potential to integrate those principles in enhancing depression awareness [18]. Thus, this study aims to propose the conceptual model of wearable persuasive multimedia to enhance awareness, particularly controllability awareness, to lower the risk of depression, especially among undergraduates.

2   The Conceptual Model: Development Process

The innards for each component of a conceptual model are determined through the implementation of content analysis. As previously discussed, [14–16, 19] has applied this kind of analysis in developing their model. For this study, the analysis involved four phases, as depicted in Fig. 1. Sections 2.1–2.4 provide the discussion of detailed activity for each phase.

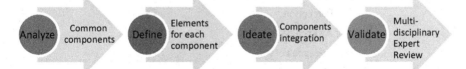

Fig. 1. Conceptual model development phases

2.1   Analyze: Common Components

Altogether, 22 studies were selected based on keywords related to persuasive multimedia in various domains and technologies and utilized persuasive or/and multimedia principles. Those criteria determine the common components and subcomponents, where both are the primary requirement of the conceptual model in enhancing controllability awareness. As displayed in Table 1, it clearly shows that most of the chosen sub-components (in bold) have a higher percentage of frequency compared to other potential sub-components.

2.2   Define: Elements for Each Sub-component

Sub-component: Persuasive, Multimedia, and Wearable Design Principles
In consequence, the previous analysis phase successfully identifies 29 persuasive and 13 multimedia design principles. Furthermore, a study by [18] also confirmed that some studies integrate both design principles. Therefore, all the persuasive multimedia studies are selected to define persuasive and multimedia principles because the effectiveness of principle integration has undergone an empirical test.

As for wearable, the user interface design was defined as an essential element because it will serve as an interface that can influence and attract users to achieve the target outcome. Therefore, all the studies that implemented user interface design were chosen in eliciting the common user interface components. Eventually, the most utilized interface design and suitable to be applied in wearable technology were considered the elements of this sub-component.

Sub-component: Controllability Awareness
The selected studies that target awareness as an outcome reported in various domains, including mental health. In psychological terms, awareness is when individuals are aware of their feelings and behaviour [20]. However, people who suffer from depression are

Table 1. Percentage of the frequency of common components and sub-components

Common components	Sub-components	Percentage of the frequency
Design principles	**Persuasive Design Principle**	**73.3**
	Wearable Design Principle	**18.8**
	Multimedia Design Principle	**45.5**
Target outcome	Behaviour	27.3
	Knowledge	9.1
	Perception	4.5
	Awareness	**36.4**
	Engagement	13.6
	Motivation	13.6
	Attitude	9.1
	Habit	4.5
User	Children	36.4
	Youth	**40.9**
	Adults	45.45
	Seniors	18.18
Technology	Computer-based	45.5
	Mobile Technology	40.9
	Wearable	**31.8**

caused by lack of controllability awareness [2]. Controllability awareness can be measured using four controllability aspects: Personal control, Shared control, Others in control, and No one in control, as stated in the Controllability Awareness Inventory (CAI) developed by [21]. [21] use the inventory to evaluate controllability awareness as a characteristic of stress tolerance. Meanwhile, [3] use it to assess the controllability awareness among schools' teachers as a predictor of effective coping in potentially traumatic stress situations after a Katyusha rocket attack. For this sub-component, controllability awareness is the most relevant element, even though it is not highlighted in any selected studies that intend to raise awareness in mental health.

Sub-component: Youth
This study will give proper attention to young adults undertaking tertiary education in Malaysian public universities, also known as university students. The consideration is due to various determinant factors of academic depression that may lead to deterioration in their academic achievement [22], may impair a relationship [23], problems in marriage, and affect their employment in the future [24]. Therefore, in identifying their emotion, the physiological symptoms such as heartbeat, respiration rate, blood pressure, Galvanic Skin Response (GSR) measurements, and other nervous system responses [25] could provide an accurate signal. Although only several selected studies used physiological

symptoms, all the studies that detect or monitor emotional changes reported measuring heart rate and heart rate variability. Thus, heart rate is the chosen element for the sub-component of the physiological parameter.

Sub-component: Wearable Technology
The behavioural, psychological, and social signals that often reflected the mental state changes [9] could be detected using the sensing technologies integrated into wearable devices. Therefore, it is crucial to identify an appropriate sensor in the wearable capable of measuring the targeted physiological parameter. For example, in detecting heart rate or heart rate variability, the selected studies utilizing wearable technology were reported using a pulse oximeter sensor to measure the symptoms.

Apart from the sensor, the other elements that need to be considered are the types of wearable as they can be divided into groups of screen-based and non-screen-based. For instance, studies that utilize smartwatches and fitness trackers can be considered as a screen-based group, while studies that use wearables such as gloves, shirts, and belts are categorized as non-screen-based. Unlike non-screen-based, users can directly access the application via the wearable screen without tethering with other devices such as smartphones. Furthermore, it is also imperative to consider the size of the screen as it will implicate the user interface design.

2.3   Ideate: Components Integration

In this phase, all the defined elements for each sub-component were integrated, forming a framework as depicted in Fig. 2. The framework was ideated based on the Generic Steps in Persuasive System Development suggested by [26], where all steps are essential in realizing an idea into reality. In the framework, many aspects are implicitly covered, including responsiveness, error-freeness, ease of access, ease of use, convenience, information quality, positive user experience, attractiveness, user loyalty, and simplicity. Those aspects need to be recognized when designing a persuasive system. However, prior to communicating the ideas to developers, precise requirements for software qualities need to be defined. Eventually, software quality checklists must be prepared to evaluate the persuasive system.

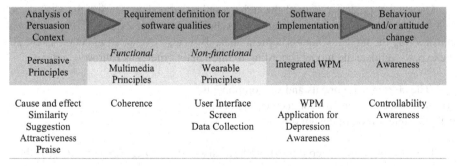

Fig. 2. The framework of Wearable Persuasive Multimedia (WPM) integration

For this study, multimedia principles are defined as functional requirements to describe how the system should behave, while wearable principles are the non-functional requirements that specify the qualities that should be owned by the system [27, 28]. Eventually, the selected persuasive principles are integrated with the system requirements and embedded in the Wearable Persuasive Multimedia application to enhance controllability awareness. Next, the framework was transferred into a conceptual model that will be explained in Sect. 3.

2.4 Validate: Multidisciplinary Expert Reviews

Finally, the conceptual model underwent a first validation process by using the multidisciplinary expert reviews method. The method was suggested by [29] and implemented in [30] to cover all the viewpoints, which are user acceptance, mobile intervention design, and persuasive design, that are required in their study. As this study will also be looking into multi-technology and human psychology, all appointed experts were among the academics and practitioners with years of experience in the related field of persuasive multimedia, wearable technology, and human psychology. The detailed information of all experts is demonstrated in Table 2.

Table 2. Experts' information

Expert	Position	Year of experience	Field	Organization
1	Academic	More than five years	Persuasive Technology, Multimedia Technology, Wearable Technology	Public university
2	Academic	More than five years	Persuasive Technology, Multimedia Technology	Public university
3	Academic	More than five years	Persuasive Technology, Multimedia Technology	Public university
4	Psychologist	More than five years	Human Psychology	Ministry of Health of Malaysia

The review process occurred through an online workshop. During the workshop, first, the researcher presents and introduces the model to the experts. The process of constructing the model, which is content analysis, is also explained in detail. Then, all the experts validate the model according to three main criteria as follow:

i)   The chosen components and subcomponents
ii) The selected elements for each component
iii) The integration of design principles

The review process continued with a discussion where experts shared their comments, feedback, and recommendation.

3   The Conceptual Model: Result and Discussion

The main issue highlighted by the experts is how the conditions are set in selecting the elements in the Design Principles component. Before the review, all the principles that at least fulfil two criteria were chosen as depicted in Table 3.

Table 3. Design principles of persuasive, wearable and multimedia technology based on 2-selected criteria

Technology	Design Principles	Criteria ☺	🕐	☑	🐍	WPM
Persuasive	Cause and effect	/		/	/	Y
	Similarity	/	/	/	/	Y
	Suggestion	/	/	/	/	Y
	Reduction	/	/			Y
	Mobile Simplicity	/			/	Y
	Attractiveness	/		/	/	Y
	Praise	/		/	/	Y
	Motivation					
	Experience					
	Cognitive					
	Emotional Appeal					
	Simulation	/	/			Y
	Social learning	/			/	Y
	Conditioning					
	Virtual rehearsal				/	
	Self-monitoring	/	/			Y
	Information quality	/			/	Y
Multimedia	Feedback	/			/	Y
	Segmentation					
	Coherence	/		/	/	Y
	Redundancy	/			/	Y
	Modality	/			/	Y
	Layout & consistency					
	Simulation					
	Navigation					
	Minimal input device					
	Personalization	/				
	Multimedia	/		/		Y
	Spatial contiguity	/			/	Y
	Temporal contiguity				/	

Table 4. Design principles of persuasive, wearable and multimedia technology based on n-selected criteria

Technology	Design Principles	Criteria				WPM			
		☺	⌚	☑	❤	1 criterion	2 criteria	3 criteria	4 criteria
Persuasive	Cause and effect	/		/	/	Y	Y	Y	
	Similarity	/	/	/	/	Y	Y	Y	Y
	Suggestion	/	/	/	/	Y	Y	Y	Y
	Reduction	/	/			Y	Y		
	Mobile Simplicity	/			/	Y	Y		
	Attractiveness	/		/	/	Y	Y	Y	
	Praise	/		/	/	Y	Y	Y	
	Motivation								
	Experience								
	Cognitive								
	Emotional Appeal								
	Simulation	/	/			Y	Y		
	Social learning	/			/	Y	Y		
	Conditioning								
	Virtual rehearsal				/	Y			
	Self-monitoring	/	/			Y	Y		
	Information quality	/			/	Y	Y		
Multimedia	Feedback	/			/	Y	Y		
	Segmentation								
	Coherence	/		/	/	Y	Y	Y	
	Redundancy	/			/	Y	Y		
	Modality	/			/	Y	Y		
	Layout & consistency								
	Simulation								
	Navigation								
	Minimal input device								
	Personalization	/				Y			
	Multimedia	/		/		Y	Y		
	Spatial contiguity	/			/	Y	Y		
	Temporal contiguity				/	Y			

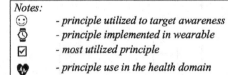

Notes:
☺   - principle utilized to target awareness
⌚   - principle implemented in wearable
☑   - most utilized principle
❤   - principle use in the health domain
Y   - Yes

However, the reviewers suggested constructing an n-criteria table, as shown in Table 4, where design principles can be appropriately selected based on the best number of selected criteria.

Consequently, the elements are chosen based on the frequency of the design principles that fulfil three-selected criteria because the number of principles is relevant to apply in the model. Moreover, more criteria in selecting the elements were considered to compensate for the shortage of probably more relevant studies. Based on experts' feedback, comments, and suggestions, the relationships among the four major components and their sub-components and their defined elements are finally expressed through the conceptual model (as depicted in Fig. 3). The proposed conceptual model is assembled based on Generic Steps in Persuasive System Development (as discussed in Sect. 2.3), comprising four main components: Design Principles, Technology, User, and Target Outcome. Every main component consists of sub-components and the selected elements. All the main components are connected according to their dependency on one another.

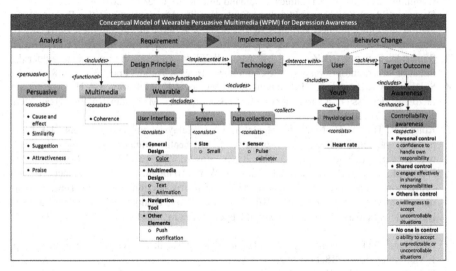

Fig. 3. Conceptual model of Wearable Persuasive Multimedia (WPM) for depression awareness

4 Conclusion

This study believes that awareness regarding the vitality of mental health problems, especially to specific target groups, can be promoted and enhanced through recent technology. In line with the plan to improve controllability awareness among university students pertinent to depression issues, an integrated model comprising wearable, persuasive, and multimedia design principles is proposed. The conceptual model is suggested due to the absence of wearable, persuasive, and multimedia design principles integration in enhancing controllability awareness in mental health-related issues. Thus, a conceptual model is constructed through a series of rigorous content analysis. Through all the processes, the main component and sub-components of the model and their elements were identified. After thorough multidisciplinary expert review sessions, the conceptual model has undergone a refinement process. Finally, the proposed conceptual model is assembled based on Generic Steps in Persuasive System Development (as discussed in Sect. 2.3), comprising four main components: Design Principles, Technology, User, and Target Outcome. The validated model is aimed to serve as a guideline by the application developers in developing a solution to enhance controllability awareness on mental health-related issues.

Acknowledgement. This research was supported by the Ministry of Education (MOE) through Fundamental Research Grant Scheme (FRGS/1/2019/ICT04/UUM/02/5).

References

1. Institute for Public Health (IPH). National Health and Morbidity Survey 2019: Non-Communicable Diseases, Healthcare Demand and Health Literacy (2019)
2. Dasgupta, M.: A Psychosocial Study of Controllability Awareness, Cognitive Emotion Regulation and Other Related Variables Across Some Selected Clinical Samples. University of Calcutta (2008)
3. Somer, E., Weitzman, A.Z., Heth, J.T.: Controllability awareness in professionals under the threat of terror: chronic versus acute community stress. J. Trauma Pract. 3(1), 1–18 (2004)
4. Suleiman, A.K., Ismadi, N.F.I., Choudhry, F.R., Munawar, K., Muhammed, A.H.: Determinant factors of depression: a survey among university students. Malaysian J. Public Heal. Med. 17(3), 97–103 (2017)
5. Kotera, Y., Ting, S.-H., Neary, S.: Mental health of Malaysian university students: UK comparison, and relationship between negative mental health attitudes, self-compassion, and resilience. High. Educ. 81(2), 403–419 (2020). https://doi.org/10.1007/s10734-020-00547-w
6. Islam, M.A., Low, W.Y., Wen, T.T., Choo, C.W.Y., Abdullah, A.: Factors associated with depression among university students in Malaysia: a cross-sectional study. In: The 2nd International Meeting of Public Health 2016 with theme "Public Health Perspective of Sustainable Development Goals: The Challenges and Opportunities in Asia-Pacific Region, pp. 415–427 (2018)
7. Robotham, D.: Do We still have a digital divide in mental health? a five-year survey follow-up. J. Med. Internet Res. 18(11) (2016
8. Burnett-Ziegler, I.E., Waldron, E.M., Hong, S., Yang, A., Wisner, K.L., Ciolino, J.D.: Accessibility and feasibility of using technology to support mindfulness practice, reduce stress and promote long term mental health. Complement. Ther. Clin. Prat. 33, 93–99 (2018)
9. Saeed, A., Tanzeem, C.: Sensing technologies for monitoring serious mental illness. IEEE Multimedia no. January–March 2018 (2018)
10. Orji, R., Moffatt, K.: Persuasive technology for health and wellness: state-of-the-art and emerging trends. Health Inform. J. 24(1), 66–91 (2018)
11. Fogg, B.J.: Persuasive Technology: Using Computers to Change What We Think and Do. Morgan Kaufmann (2003)
12. Fogg, B.J., Cuellar, G., Danielson, D.: Motivating, influencing, and persuading users. In: Jacko, J.A., Sears, A. (eds.) The human-computer interaction handbook, pp. 358–370. Lawrence Erlbaum Associate Inc, Hillsdale, NJ, USA (2007)
13. Zulkifli, A.N., Ahmad, M., Bakar, A.J.A., Mat, C.R., Noor, M.N.: Interactive persuasive learning for the elderly: a conceptual model interactive persuasive learning for the elderly: a conceptual model. In: 1st International Conference on Educational Studies (ICES-2015), pp. 1–12 (2015)

14. Ibrahim, N.: Cnceptual Design Model for Youth Personal Decision Aid. Universiti Utara Malaysia (201)7

15. Ahmad, S.Z.: A Conceptual Model of Interactive Computer Assisted Learning for Low Achieving Primary School Student. Universiti Utara Malaysia (2017)

16. Sarif, S.M.: Conceptual Design Model of Computerized Personal-Decision Aid (ComPDA). Universiti Utara Malaysia (2011)

17. Mutalib, A.A.: Conceptual Design of Reality Learning Media (RLM) Model Based on Entertaining and Fun Constructs, p. 294 (2009)

18. Mazlan, U.H., Sarif, S.M., Abdul Salam, S.N., Faisal Mohamed, N.F.: A review of persuasive multimedia principles in wearable technology for enhanced awareness depression: opportunities for consolidation. In: e-Proceedings: Creative Humanities International Conference (CHiC 2020), pp. 55–63 (2020)

19. Mutalib, A.A.: Conceptual design of Reality Learning Media (RLM) model based on entertaining and fun constructs (2009)

20. Dohalit, M.L., Salam, A.S.N., Mutalib, A.A.: A Review on Persuasive Technology (PT) Strategy in Awareness Study. vol. 9, no. September (2016)

21. Heth, J.T., Somer, E.: Characterizing stress tolerance: 'controllability awareness' and its relationship to perceived stress and reported health. Pers. Individ. Dif. **33**, 883–895 (2002)

22. Stewart-Brown, S., et al.: The health of students in institutes of higher education: an important and neglected public health problem? J. Public Health Med. **22**(4), 492–499 (2000)

23. Ali, B.S., Rahbar, M.H., Naeem, S., Tareen, A.L., Gui, A., Samad, L.: Prevalence of and factors associated with anxiety and depression among women in a lower middle class semi-urban community of Karachi, Pakistan. J. Pak. Med. Assoc. **52**(11), 513–517 (2002)

24. Eisenberg, D., Gollust, S.E., Golberstein, E., Hefner, J.L.: Prevalence and correlates of depression, anxiety, and suicidality among university students. Am. J. Orthopsych. **77**(4), 534–542 (2007)

25. Balters, S., Steinert, M.: Capturing emotion reactivity through physiology measurement as a foundation for affective engineering in engineering design science and engineering practices. J. Intell. Manuf. **28**(7), 1585–1607 (2015). https://doi.org/10.1007/s10845-015-1145-2

26. Oinas-Kukkonen, H., Harjumaa, M.: Persuasive systems design: key issues, process model, and system features. Commun. Assoc. Inf. Syst. **24**(1), 485–500 (2009)

27. Robertson, S., Robertson, J.: Mastering the Requirements Process. Addison-Wesley London, Upper Saddle River, N.J (2006)

28. Sommerville, I., Sawyer, S.: Requirements Engineering: A Good Practice Guide. John Wiley, Chichester (1997)

29. Bass, L.J., Gornostaev, J., Unger, C. (eds.): EWHCI 1993. LNCS, vol. 753. Springer, Heidelberg (1993). https://doi.org/10.1007/3-540-57433-6

30. Chang, T.-R., Kaasinen, E., Kaipainen, K.: Persuasive design in mobile applications for mental well-being: multidisciplinary expert review. In: Godara, B., Nikita, K.S. (eds.) LNICST 61, pp. 154–162. Springer, Cham (2013). https://doi.org/10.1007/978-3-642-37893-5_18

Information Systems – Information Retrieval

A Comparative Study of Data Mining Techniques Applied to Renal-Cell Carcinomas

Ana Duarte[1] 📵, Hugo Peixoto[2(✉)] 📵, and José Machado[2] 📵

[1] University of Minho, Campus Gualtar, Braga, Portugal
[2] Centro Algoritmi, University of Minho, Campus Gualtar, Braga, Portugal
hpeixoto@di.uminho.pt

Abstract. Despite being one of the deadliest diseases and the enormous evolution in fighting it, the best methods to predict kidney cancer, namely Renal-Cell Carcinomas (RCC), are not well-known. One of the solutions to accelerate the current knowledge about RCC is through the use of Data Mining techniques based on patients' personal and clinical data. Therefore, it is crucial to understand which techniques are the most suitable to extract knowledge about this disease. In this paper, we followed the CRISP-DM methodology to simulate different techniques to determine the ones with the best predictive performance. For this purpose, we used a dataset of 821 records of RCC patients, obtained from The Cancer Genome Atlas. The present work tests different Data Mining techniques, that can be used to predict the 5-year life expectancy of patients with renal cancer and to predict the number of days to death for patients who have a life expectancy of less than 5 years. The results obtained demonstrated that the best algorithm for estimating the vital status at 5 years was Random Forest. This algorithm presented an accuracy of 87.65% and an AUROC of 0.931. For the prediction of days to death, the best performance was obtained with the k-Nearest Neighbors algorithm with a root mean square error of 354.6 days. The work suggested that Data Mining techniques can help to understand the influence of various risk factors on the life expectancy of patients with RCC.

Keywords: Renal-Cell Carcinoma · Data Mining · Survival · Life expectancy · RapidMiner

1 Introduction

On a global scale, cancer is one of the major concerns of public health authorities. One of the most common type is kidney cancer, which causes approximately 430,000 new cases per year and corresponds to the 15th deadliest cancer worldwide [1]. The most representative form of kidney cancer is Renal-Cell Carcinoma (RCC), which accounts for about 90% of total cases, and refers to any malignant tumour that originates from the renal epithelium. This type of disease is divided into several histologic subtypes that have different specific characteristics. Clear-cell RCC (ccRCC), papillary RCC (pRCC) and chromophobe RCC (chRCC) are the most typical forms, and the other subtypes

© ICST Institute for Computer Sciences, Social Informatics and Telecommunications Engineering 2022
Published by Springer Nature Switzerland AG 2022. All Rights Reserved
S. Spinsante et al. (Eds.): HealthyIoT 2021, LNICST 432, pp. 53–62, 2022.
https://doi.org/10.1007/978-3-030-99197-5_5

represent only a residual proportion of the total incidence. The predominant subtype is ccRCC (≈75% of the total), followed by pRCC (≈10%) and chRCC (≈5%) [2–4].

The Tumour Node Metastasis (TNM) staging system is the most widely used tool for classifying malignant tumours, including RCC. According to the system's terminology, T refers to the size and extent of the primary tumour and indicates whether it has grown into nearby areas; N whether the tumour has spread to nearby lymph nodes; and M refers to metastasis, that is, if the cancer has spread to other parts of the body [5, 6]. In order to go into more detail about RCC, each of these letters can be divided into different groups, as summarized in Table 1.

Table 1. RCC classification according to the TNM staging system [5].

TNM	Meaning	Types
T1	Tumour is only in the kidney with 7 cm or less	T1a → greatest dimension <4 cm T1b → greatest dimension 4–7 cm
T2	Tumour is only in the kidney with more than 7 cm	T2a → greatest dimension 7–10 cm T2b → greatest dimension >10 cm
T3	Tumour has spread into major veins or perinephric tissues	T3a → has grown into the renal vein or its branches, or has invaded perirenal and/or renal sinus fat but not beyond Gerota fascia T3b → has grown into inferior vena cava T3c → has grown into vena cava above the diaphragm or has invaded the wall of the vena cava
T4	Tumour has proliferated to areas beyond Gerota fascia	
N	Tumour has spread to regional lymph nodes	NX → regional lymph nodes cannot be evaluated N0 → no regional lymph node metastasis N1 → metastasis in regional lymph node(s)
M	Presence or absence of distant metastasis	M0 → no distant metastasis M1 → the cancer has spread to distant organs

Medical knowledge about RCC has made great strides, and the main risk factors for developing the disease are already well-established. Smoking, physical inactivity, diabetes, hypertension, obesity, family history, age, gender, and ethnicity are some of the factors that have an impact on increasing the likelihood of developing RCC [7]. The steady increase in knowledge in this field has led to more sophisticated diagnostic techniques, resulting in a significant improvement in the 5-year overall survival rate, which has risen from 57% to 74% in recent years [3].

The 5-year survival rate is a widely used indicator to measure the severity of cancer and represents the percentage of patients who are still alive after a 5-year period since the diagnosis of the disease. For kidney cancer specifically, the 5-year survival rate is usually estimated by considering only the locations to which the cancer has spread, as shown in Fig. 1. The information illustrated in Fig. 1 is based on SEER database [8].

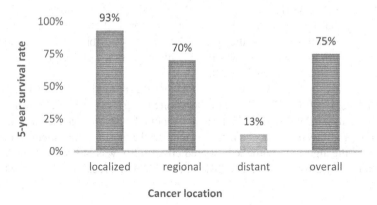

Fig. 1. 5-year survival rate according to the tumor's location.

However, the estimate of the 5-year survival rate could be improved by including more features beyond tumour location, and by considering the interactions that exist between them. In order to achieve a more accurate estimate of 5-year survival rate, we can use Data Mining (DM) techniques combining multiple features. The two main advantages of these techniques are the possibility of developing complex predictive models that are close to reality and the fact that they do not require long studies that consume many resources. DM techniques can be easily adapted to predict the survival estimate for different time periods with small adjustments to the models in a relatively simple way.

In this context, the present work aims to compare the predictive capacity of different DM algorithms to determine the best suited models to predict whether a given patient has a life expectancy of more or less than 5 years and, if less, to estimate the expected days of life.

The paper is organized into five main sections. This first section gives a brief overview of kidney cancer, RCC and DM techniques. The second section presents some related work, and the third section describes the materials and methods. Finally, Sect. 4 analyses and discusses the obtained results and Sect. 5 summarizes the main conclusions and some possible future work.

2   Related Work

In recent years, some approaches have been proposed in the literature to investigate the use of DM techniques in kidney diseases. At this level, in 2014, Zeenia Jagga and Dinesh Gupta used J48, Random Forest (RF), Sequential Minimal Optimization (SMO) and Naïve Bayes (NB) techniques to identify whether a kidney cancer is at an "early stage" (stage i or stage II) or at a "late stage" (stage iii or stage iv). The dataset used comprised a total of 62 genes and the results obtained demonstrated that the RF algorithm presented the best predictive values, with a sensitivity of 89%, an accuracy of 77%, and an Area Under Receivers Operating Curve (AUROC) of 0.8 [9].

In its turn, in 2019, El-Houssainy A. Rady and Ayman S. Anwarb tested the Probabilistic Neural Networks (PNN), Multilayer Perceptron (MLP), Support Vector Machine (SVM) and Radial Base Function (RBF) algorithms for predicting the stage of chronic kidney disease. For this purpose, they used a dataset of 24 attributes and concluded that the algorithm with the best values was PNN, with an accuracy of 99.7%, a precision of 98.7% and an F-Measure of 99.4% [10].

More recently, in 2020, Aranuwa Felix Ola tested J48, Logistic Model Tree (LMT), M5P, REPTree, Hoeffding Tree (VFDT), Decision Stump (DS) and RF algorithms using Weka. The analysed data contained information about the patient's gender, age, lifestyle, gender and hereditary disorder, chemical and industrial exposure, and patient complaints. In this study, the algorithm with the best predictive ability was J48, with an accuracy of 74.7%, an F-Measure of 61.4%, a precision of 68.7% and a recall of 71.4% [11].

3   Materials and Methods

The dataset used for the present study was obtained from the Genomic Data Commons of the National Institutes of Health (NIH) of the USA, which provides clinical and genomic data from cancer research programs for research purposes [12]. The dataset includes data from The Cancer Genome Atlas (TCGA) projects – TCGA-KIRC, TCGA-KIRP and TCGA-KICH – and relates to patients with RCC. TCGA selects different cancers for study which have poor prognosis capacity and a high public health impact [13].

The data processing and the construction of the predictive models were performed using RapidMiner software, following the Cross Industry Standard Process for Data Mining (CRISP-DM) methodology [14]. This methodology enumerates a series of steps that enable the implementation of data mining projects from situations in real context [15]. In the case of present work, we followed the CRISP-DM methodology to create the DM models for each of the proposed objectives: Determine whether a patient is likely to be alive 5 years after the diagnosis of RCC and predict life expectancy in the cases where the prognosis is worse.

3.1   Data Preprocessing

The original dataset consists of 821 records and 154 personal and clinical attributes, including *vital_status* and *days_to_death* attributes. Based on these two parameters, it is possible to apply different DM algorithms to respond to the outlined objectives.

At this stage, the raw data were treated in order to:

- Check their consistency by analysing redundant attributes – The original dataset contained some redundant attributes, such as age in years and age in days. In these cases, the inconsistent records were removed.
- Replace missing data with existing redundant attributes – In the case of existing redundant fields, the missing values were replaced by the values of the duplicated columns.

- Eliminate irrelevant columns for the DM process; columns without any values filled in; or fields that refer to duplicate/redundant data.

Since the dataset contained redundant pathological and clinical data, the latter columns were eliminated as pathological data are more reliable. In case of inconsistencies, the priority was given to pathological data. If there were missing values in the pathological data, those cells were replaced with the corresponding clinical values.

At the end of these steps, the attributes were reduced to the following 11: *age_at_index, ajcc_pathologic_m, ajcc_pathologic_n, ajcc_pathologic_t, ajcc_pathologic_stage, gender, primary_diagnosis, prior_malignancy, race, days_to_death and vital_status.*

Considering the classification of the TNM staging system, the consistency of the data was checked using the following rules [5]:

- If Stage I then M0, N0, T1
- If Stage II then M0, N0, T2
- If Stage III then (M0, N1, T1 or T2) or (M0, any N, T3)
- If Stage IV then (M0, any N, T4) or (M1, any N, any T)

Moreover, these rules also allowed the derivation of some missing values related to M, N, T, and stage. For example, for the records referring to stage I or II with missing values in *ajcc*_pathologic_*n*, we have replaced those missing values by N0. Afterwards, since *ajcc_pathologic_stage* contained some missing values that could not be inferred by the rules, the corresponding rows were removed. In addition, some records contained the non-specific histological term "renal cell carcinoma, NOS" in the *primary_diagnosis* column [16]. These values were replaced by the most common specific type of RCC ("clear cell adenocarcinoma, NOS").

The basic statistics of the numeric and nominal attributes after the data preprocessing are presented in Table 2 and Table 3, respectively.

Table 2. Summary statistics for numerical attributes

Numeric attribute	Min	Max	Average	Standard deviation	Missing values
age_at_index	17	90	60.341	12.393	0.37%
days_to_death	0	3615	910.129	731.614	74.97%

From the data analysis, it can be observed that the "alive" and "dead" values of the class label *vital_status* were not balanced. In order to obtain more balanced data, we have simulated the application of different methodologies, including SMOTE, but the best option was to perform a simple oversampling of duplication of records with respect to the "dead" value to improve the system's performance [17, 18]. After this procedure, the number of "dead" records was increased to 606.

Table 3. Summary statistics for nominal attributes

Nominal attribute	Values	Number of records	Missing values
ajcc_pathologic_m	M0/M1	712/90	0.12%
ajcc_pathologic_n	N0/N1/N2	655/40/6	12.70%
ajcc_pathologic_stage	Stage I/II Stage III/IV	433/96 179/95	0.00%
ajcc_pathologic_t	T1/T1a/T1b T2/T2a/T2b T3/T3a/T3b/T3c T4	46/229/164 81/18/15 14/158/62/2 14	0.00%
Gender	Male/Female	536/267	0.00%
primary_diagnosis	CCA/PA/RCC	468/262/59	1.74%
prior_malignancy	Yes/No	113/690	0.00%
Race	White/Black nr/asian/native	653/116 18/14/2	0.00%
vital_status	Alive/Dead	601/202	0.00%

3.2 Data Cleansing

After inserting the preprocessed dataset into RapidMiner, we built a block called "Data Cleansing", which consists of several processes that perform the following additional data treatment operations:

- The records of patients who died that were associated with "0" in the *days_to_death* field were removed.
- The missing values in *days_to_death*, *primary_diagnosis* and *age_at_index* attributes were replaced by *zero*, *"Clear cell adenocarcinoma, NOS"* and by the mean age, respectively.
- The records were filtered to include only patients who died within 5 years of the diagnosis date (*days_to_death* $<= 1825$), and patients under 75 years (*age_at_index* $<= 75$).
- Records containing outliers were removed.

Depending on whether the purpose of the prediction is to classify the vital status as "alive" or "dead" or to estimate the number of days until death, the system then performs different operations. In the first case, the *days_to_death* column was removed and in the second case, the nominal attributes were converted to numeric values and the rows related to the vital status "alive" were removed.

3.3 Modeling and Validation

To model the problem, we followed 2 different methodologies, depending on the expected target. Target 1 aims to determine the vital status of a patient 5 years after the diagnosis of the disease. Target 2 intends to estimate the life expectancy for patients who are not expected to survive longer than 5 years. For each of these objectives, we tested different DM techniques in order to obtain reliable predictive models. The techniques that led to the best results were:

- DM techniques for Target 1 = {Random Forest, Rule Induction, Generalized Linear Model, Logistic Regression, k-Nearest Neighbors}
- DM techniques for Target 2 = {Linear Regression, Generalized Linear Model, Neural Net, Deep Learning, k-Nearest Neighbors}

For the construction of the predictive models, for the training and validation phases, a 10-fold cross-validation approach was used for target 1, and a leave-one-out cross-validation was used for target 2. In this step, the parameters were optimized to obtain the highest values for accuracy, precision, recall and AUROC, in the case of target 1, and the lowest Root Mean Square Error (RMSE) in the case of target 2.

Accuracy represents the percentage of correct predictions, precision refers to the percentage of positive predictions (dead) that were correctly identified, and recall indicates the percentage of positive cases that were correctly identified. On the other hand, the AUROC indicator provides information about the quality and robustness of the model and the RMSE measures the deviations of the prediction errors.

In the specific case of medical predictions, it is more important to minimize false negatives than false positives. False negatives, in this context, correspond to the patients who died but which the algorithm predicts to be "alive" and false positives correspond to the patients who survived but that were predicted to be "dead". A situation in which a healthy person is falsely identified as sick can be corrected by complementary testing. However, if a sick person is falsely diagnosed as healthy, this false prognosis may delay the treatments needed to combat the disease. Thus, for target 1 is important to obtain high recall values. In the case of target 2, the performance of the models was analysed considering the indicator RMSE.

In addition to checking the performance of the models, it is also important to analyse whether they are overfitted or not. In order to test the models, the data were split into two subsets: one with 80% of the data for training and validation, and a second subset with 20% of the data for an independent test of the models.

4 Results and Discussion

To select the algorithm that best fits each target, we compared the values of the main performance indicators obtained during the train and test phases. For the classification of the patients' vital status, these values are summarized in Table 4.

As indicated in Table 4, the models have similar measurements in both training and testing phases. Therefore, it was concluded that the created models were not overfitted. Regarding the ability to predict the patients' vital status, the technique that presented the best results was RF, which achieved high values for accuracy (87.65%), precision (82.36%), recall (92.23%) and AUROC (0.931) and an acceptable runtime. Some of the considered parameters for this algorithm were 40 trees, "gini-index" criterion, and

Table 4. Performance of algorithms in classification process (alive/dead).

Algorithm		Accuracy (%)	Precision (%)	Recall (%)	AUROC	Runtime* (ms)
Random Forest	Train	87.65	82.36	92.23	0.931	345
	Test	86.60	80.61	91.86	0.949	
Rule Induction	Train	80.82	78.18	78.90	0.838	1139
	Test	77.32	75.00	73.26	0.822	
Generalized Linear Model	Train	78.88	79.43	64.39	0.800	198
	Test	76.92	69.81	64.91	0.794	
Logistic Regression	Train	76.70	78.83	65.83	0.821	149
	Test	72.68	73.85	57.14	0.816	
k-Nearest Neighbors	Train	79.29	81.03	70.79	0.888	115
	Test	74.74	73.42	67.44	0.842	

* Total runtime for training and testing phases calculated with Jackhammer extension.

a "maximal depth" of 15. The obtained performance metrics enable to consider that RF is suitable for determining life expectancy at 5 years and can be used as a complement to medical diagnosis.

For the analysis of the life expectancy estimation, the values obtained in terms of RMSE are illustrated in Fig. 2.

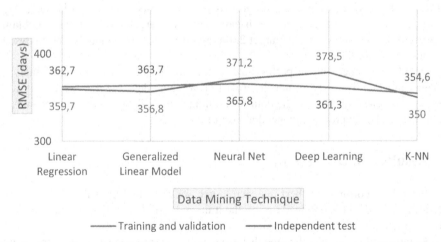

Fig. 2. Comparison of the RMSE between the training and testing phases for each DM technique.

Despite the high margin of error found for each algorithm (~1 year), it is possible to get a general idea of the number of years of life that are expected. From this point of view, the best performance values were obtained using the k-Nearest Neighbors (k-NN) technique, which presented a RMSE of 354.6 days, and the Deep Learning (DL) technique, which presented a RMSE of 361.3 days. In turn, the Linear Regression (LR) technique presented a RMSE of 362.7 days. This technique has the advantage of providing an easy-to-understand and easy-to-use prediction mechanism that can be used for an initial assessment of the severity of the disease. The equation obtained by the LR algorithm was:

$$days\_to\_death = 86.317 \times ajcc\_patho \log ic\_n$$
$$- 129.988 \times ajcc\_patho \log ic\_stage + 775.348$$

This equation was obtained considering only the *ajcc_pathologic_n* and *ajcc_pathologic_stage* attributes, since they were the only ones that had a p-value of less than 0.05, which makes them the most important parameters for predicting life expectancy. The p-values obtained were 0.079 for *age_at_index*, 0.048 for *ajcc_pathologic_n*, 0.001 for *ajcc_pathologic_stage*, 0.124 for *ajcc_pathologic_t*, 0.512 for *gender*, 0.991 for *primary_diagnosis*, and 0.619 for *prior_malignancy*.

In terms of execution times, the k-NN and LR algorithms were the fastest with 19 and 63 ms, respectively. On the other hand, DL and NN were the slowest algorithms with 3027 and 844 ms, respectively.

5   Conclusions and Future Work

This paper aimed to identify the most suitable DM techniques and their parameters for predictions related to RCC. The DM techniques used allow the construction of complex prediction models that take into account the influence of multiple attributes simultaneously. The constructed models allow predicting whether a given patient has a life expectancy of at least 5 years and, in the worst scenarios, they allow calculating the patients' life expectancy. These models can be used as a valuable tool to complement medical diagnosis.

By simulating different techniques and optimizing their parameters, we have verified that the RF algorithm has a high efficiency to characterize the vital status of RCC patients at five years. On the other hand, the LR algorithm provides a simple and easy to understand mechanism to calculate the life expectancy of RCC patients, with a margin of error of about 1 year.

Although the present study is based on real data, it would be interesting for future work to replicate the experience with a larger dataset, also including more columns corresponding to other important risk factors, such as genes, workplaces exposures, or body mass indexes. A larger dataset could even contribute to improve the predictive models.

Acknowledgements. This work is funded by "FCT—Fundação para a Ciência e Tecnologia" within the R&D Units Project Scope: UIDB/00319/2020.

References

1. Sung, H., et al.: Global cancer statistics 2020: GLOBOCAN estimates of incidence and mortality worldwide for 36 cancers in 185 countries. CA. Cancer J. Clin. **71**, 209–249 (2021). https://doi.org/10.3322/caac.21660
2. Hsieh, J.J., et al.: Renal cell carcinoma. Nat. Rev. Dis. Prim. **3**, 1–19 (2017). https://doi.org/10.1038/nrdp.2017.9
3. Choueiri, T.K., Motzer, R.J.: Systemic therapy for metastatic renal-cell carcinoma. N. Engl. J. Med. **376**, 354–366 (2017)
4. Dizman, N., Philip, E.J., Pal, S.K.: Genomic profiling in renal cell carcinoma. Nat. Rev. Nephrol. **16**, 435–451 (2020). https://doi.org/10.1038/s41581-020-0301-x
5. Brierley, J.D., Gospodarowicz, M.K., Wittekind, C. (eds.): TNM Classification of Malignant Tumours. Wiley Blackwell (2017)
6. National Cancer Institute: Cancer Staging. https://www.cancer.gov/about-cancer/diagnosis-staging/staging. Accessed 08 June 2021
7. Scelo, G., Larose, T.L.: Epidemiology and risk factors for kidney cancer. J. Clin. Oncol. **36**, 3574–3581 (2018). https://doi.org/10.1200/JCO.2018.79.1905
8. American Cancer Society: Survival Rates for Kidney Cancer. https://www.cancer.org/cancer/kidney-cancer/detection-diagnosis-staging/survival-rates.html. Accessed 08 June 2021
9. Jagga, Z., Gupta, D.: Classification models for clear cell renal carcinoma stage progression, based on tumor RNAseq expression trained supervised machine learning algorithms. BMC Proc. **8**, 1–7 (2014). https://doi.org/10.1186/1753-6561-8-S6-S2
10. Rady, E.-H.A., Anwar, A.S.: Prediction of kidney disease stages using data mining algorithms. Inf. Med. Unlocked. **15**, 100178 (2019). https://doi.org/10.1016/j.imu.2019.100178
11. Ola, A.F.: A model for prediction of kidney cancer using data analytics technique. Am. J. Data Min. Knowl. Discov. **5**, 27–36 (2020). https://doi.org/10.11648/j.ajdmkd.20200502.12
12. Grossman, R.L., et al.: Toward a shared vision for cancer genomic data. N. Engl. J. Med. **375**, 1109–1112 (2016). https://doi.org/10.1056/nejmp1607591
13. National Cancer Institute: TCGA Cancers Selected for Study. https://www.cancer.gov/about-nci/organization/ccg/research/structural-genomics/tcga/studied-cancers. Accessed 17 June 2021
14. RapidMiner. https://rapidminer.com/. Accessed 07 May 2021
15. Morais, A., Peixoto, H., Coimbra, C., Abelha, A., Machado, J.: Predicting the need of neonatal resuscitation using data mining. In: Procedia Computer Science, pp. 571–576. Elsevier B.V. (2017). https://doi.org/10.1016/j.procs.2017.08.287
16. Dickie, L., Johnson, C., Adams, S., Negoita, S.: Solid Tumor Rules. National Cancer Institute, Rockville, MD (2020)
17. Chawla, N.V., Bowyer, K.W., Hall, L.O., Kegelmeyer, W.P.: SMOTE: synthetic minority over-sampling technique. J. Artif. Intell. Res. **16**, 321–357 (2002). https://doi.org/10.1613/jair.953
18. Peixoto, C., Peixoto, H., Machado, J., Abelha, A., Santos, M.F.: Iron value classification in patients undergoing continuous ambulatory peritoneal dialysis using data mining. In: Proceedings of the 4th International Conference on Information and Communication Technologies for Ageing Well and e-Health (ICT4AWE), pp. 285–290. SCITEPRESS (2018). https://doi.org/10.5220/0006820802850290

Predicting Diabetes Disease in the Female Adult Population, Using Data Mining

Carolina Marques[1] , Vasco Ramos[1] , Hugo Peixoto[2]([⊠]) ,
and José Machado[2]

[1] University of Minho, Campus Gualtar, Braga, Portugal
[2] Centro Algoritmi, University of Minho, Campus Gualtar, Braga, Portugal
hpeixoto@di.uminho.pt

Abstract. The aim of this study is to predict, through data mining, the incidence of diabetes disease in the Pima Female Adult Population. Diabetes is a chronic disease that occurs either when the pancreas does not produce enough insulin or when the body cannot effectively use the insulin it produces and is a major cause of blindness, kidney failure, heart attacks, stroke and lower limb amputation. The information collected from this population combined with the data mining techniques, may help to detect earlier the presence of this decease. To achieve the best possible ML model, this work uses the CRISP-DM methodology and compares the results of five ML models (Logistic Regression, Naive Bayes, Random Forest, Gradient Boosted Trees and k-NN) obtained from two different datasets (originated from two different data preparation strategies). The study shows that the most promising model as k-NN, which produced results of 90% of accuracy and also 90% of F1 Score, in the most realistic evaluation scenario.

Keywords: Data mining · Diabetes · CRISP-DM · Classification · ML models

1 Introduction

This paper has the purpose of diagnostically predict whether or not a patient has diabetes, considering certain variables, using Data Mining techniques with the help of RapidMiner[1].

Regarding its content, this article includes five sections. After the Introduction, the second section - Background and Related Work - presents a brief description of diabetes disease followed by previous studies and papers on this subject. The third section, Methodology, describes the applied CRISP-DM processes, which includes: business and data understanding, data preparation, modeling and evaluation. Section four presents the analysis and discussion of both

---

[1] https://rapidminer.com.

© ICST Institute for Computer Sciences, Social Informatics and Telecommunications Engineering 2022
Published by Springer Nature Switzerland AG 2022. All Rights Reserved
S. Spinsante et al. (Eds.): HealthyIoT 2021, LNICST 432, pp. 63–73, 2022.
https://doi.org/10.1007/978-3-030-99197-5_6

the achieved results and the underlying work that was required to achieve those results. Finally, the last section addresses the conclusions that were possible to be drawn and and future work and improvements that could improve the present work.

2   Background and Related Work

2.1   Diabetes

Diabetes is a chronic disease that occurs either when the pancreas does not produce enough insulin or when the body cannot effectively use the insulin[2] it produces. Hyperglycaemia, or raised blood sugar, is a common effect of uncontrolled diabetes and over time leads to serious damage to many of the body's systems, especially the nerves and blood vessels.

About 422 million people worldwide have diabetes, the majority living in low-and middle-income countries, and 1.6 million deaths are directly attributed to diabetes each year. Both the number of cases and the prevalence of diabetes have been steadily increasing over the past few decades. Diabetes of all types can lead to complications in many parts of the body and can increase the overall risk of dying prematurely. Possible complications include kidney failure, leg amputation, vision loss and nerve damage. Adults with diabetes also have two- to three-fold increased risk of heart attacks and strokes. In pregnancy, poorly controlled diabetes increases the risk of fetal death and other complications, [1].

Early diagnosis can be accomplished through relatively inexpensive blood testing, [1].

2.2   Related Work

Data Mining is defined as the process of discovering patterns in data. The patterns discovered must be meaningful in order to lead to some advantage. Useful patterns allow us to make nontrivial predictions on new data, [2,3]. With computerized technology, content and structure started to change very fast in the health sector. Provided health services have to be fast, accurate, qualified and also have to meet the required needs. In order to achieve these goals, healthcare professionals need to have the most accurate and updated information and use this information as a relevant factor in their decision support systems, [4].

Effective use of healthcare data is made possible by data mining, which allows to extract relevant and valuable knowledge from large volumes of data. In healthcare, data mining is used to predict various diseases and to help doctors diagnose, [5–7].

Furthermore, the application of Data-Mining techniques which help to create a streamlined pipeline that includes all relevant phases of this type of work (data analysis, preparation, model development and application, results evaluation,

---

[2] Insulin is a hormone that regulates blood sugar.

and deployment) and allows for a simpler process of review, improvement and comparison, [8, 9].

In [10], the study proposed to identify and classify the presence of diabetes diseases by applying data mining techniques. The dataset contained 520 instances, each having 17 attributes. Seven different classification algorithm including Bayes Network, Naïve Bayes, J48, Random Tree, Random Forest, k-NN and SVM were studied on the dataset. Obtained results indicated that k-NN performed the highest accuracy with 98.07%, being the best method to identify and classify diabetes diseases on the studied dataset. This work also presented interesting topics on how to clean and augment data, both in quantity and quality.

In [11], the study proposed a hybrid prediction model comprised of two different algorithms: the improved K-means algorithm and the logistic regression algorithm, which was based on data mining techniques for predicting type 2 *diabetes mellitus* (T2DM). The main problems trying to be solved were: improve the accuracy of the prediction model, and make the model adaptive to more than one dataset. Some previous studies have developed models with the same premise as the one for this paper, so the goal was to later compare the paper's results to those from this other papers. The dataset used on this paper was the same used on the present study (The Pima Indians Diabetes Dataset). The obtained results were compared to the results of the already mentioned previous studies and showed that the model attained a 3.04% higher accuracy of prediction (the accuracy was around 94%) than the ones used for comparison. Moreover, the model ensured that the dataset quality is sufficient. As a result, the model was shown to be useful in the realistic health management of diabetes.

3 Methodology

The data used in this work was originally provided by the **National Institute of Diabetes and Digestive and Kidney Diseases**, and has the purpose of diagnostically predict whether or not a patient has diabetes, based on some diagnostic measurements and medical indicators. The dataset is available at Pima Indians Diabetes Database - Kaggle.

Regarding the Data Mining process, this work will apply the Cross Industry Standard Process for Data Mining (CRISP-DM) Methodology, which is an hierarchical and iterative process model with six phases that naturally describes the data science life cycle. Those six phases are: **Business Understanding, Data Understanding, Data Preparation, Modeling, Evaluation** and **Deployment**, [12–14]. This process methodology was chosen due to its large set of advantages such as standardization of applied processes which makes the whole approach easily replicable, clear evaluation metrics and methods, clear structure of what to study and analyze which increases the changes of success and, finally, the possibility of applying Data Mining models in real scenarios, [15].

3.1 Business Understanding

The purpose of this study, as stated earlier, is to diagnostically predict whether or not a patient has diabetes, considering characteristics such as insulin level, plasma glucose concentration, blood pressure, skin thickness, among others. It is also relevant to point out that this study is focused on a very specific population: all patients are females, at least 21 years old, of Pima Indian heritage.

3.2 Data Understanding

The dataset used for this study, as stated earlier, consists of information regarding women of, at least, 21 years old from the Pima Indian community. It has 768 instances and each instance has 8 attributes and one more column with the respective class.

- **Pregnancies**: Number of times pregnant;
- **Glucose**: Plasma glucose concentration a 2 h in an oral glucose tolerance test;
- **Blood Pressure**: Diastolic blood pressure (mm/Hg);
- **Skin Thickness**: Triceps skin fold thickness (mm);
- **Insulin**: 2-Hour serum insulin (mu U/ml);
- **BMI**: Body mass index $(weight\_in\_kg/(height\_in\_m)^2)$;
- **DPB (Diabetes Pedigree Function)**: Diabetes pedigree function;
- **Age**: Age (in years);
- **Outcome**: Class variable that specifies if tested positive for diabetes (0 or 1): 0 if YES, 1 if NO.

For a better understanding of each attribute, the Table 1 was created. It shows the number of missing values, the minimum and maximum value, the average and standard deviation of each attribute.

Table 1. Attribute description.

Attribute	Missing	Min	Max	Avg	Std. dev.
Pregnancies	0	0	17	3.8450	3.369
Glucose	5	0	199	120.894	31.973
Blood pressure	35	0	122	69.105	19.356
Skin thickness	227	0	99	20.536	15.952
Insulin	374	0	846	79.799	115.244
BMI	11	0	67.1	31.992	7.884
DPB	0	0.078	3.420	0.472	0.3315
Age	0	21	81	33.241	11.760

The class variable (outcome) has two different values: YES or NO. Figure 1 shows the data distribution regarding the outcome class that has 268 instances

Distribution of Outcome (class)

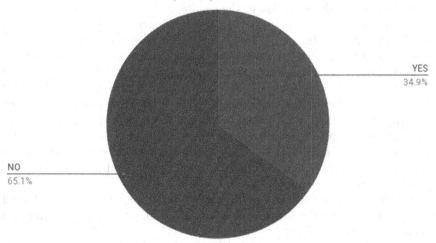

Fig. 1. Distribution of outcome (class)

of YES (34.9%) and 500 instances of NO (65.1%), which means that almost 35% of the cases indeed tested positive for diabetes and the remaining cases didn't.

The visualization of Fig. 1 clearly shows that the distribution of examples across the class Outcome is biased, having a big majority of the instances classified as NO. Having imbalanced or skewed data jeopardizes the ML models that will have poor predictive performance, specifically for the minority class.

3.3 Data Preparation

First Approach
Using the insight gained in the previous phase, the first step to clean the dataset was to map the missing values (that were described as zeros) to NaN values and remove all the instances that had missing values. After that, the dataset was normalized to values between 0 and 1 so that it was possible to find and remove the outliers more accurately. The next step is related to the fact that the dataset is skewed, so the dataset was oversampled using replication techniques over the existing data in order to balance the proportion of positive and negative instances for the diabetes test, increasing the number of instances associated with the presence of diabetes to approximate the number of negative examples. The last step was to shuffle the obtained dataset to ensure randomization in the process.

Second Approach
Being that the first approach was more focused on achieving high predicting results, the obtained dataset was not truly representative of the problem, therefore not reliable. Thus, it was decided to create an alternative approach more

focused on producing a credible and representative dataset, taking into consideration the possible deterioration of the results.

The first approach followed the strategy of removing all the instances that had missing values, whether this new methodology followed the strategy of removing the attribute with more missing values. In the dataset there were two main attributes that had missing values: *insulin*, with 374 instances (49% of all instances) and *skin thickness*, with 227 (29% of all instances). Removing both columns would reduce significantly the number of attributes (would only have 6) and the dataset itself, which would originate a poorer and more error-prone dataset. Hence, in order to create a compromise and keep the maximum number of instances while discarding a big majority of missing values, it was decided to remove only one of those two attributes: *insulin*, which, as already said, had the highest percentage of missing values.

From this point forward, the same steps of the first approach were followed, i.e., normalization, outlier identification and removal, oversampling to fix data imbalance and data shuffling.

As a final note, in both approaches the final dataset had roughly 1250 instances, with a similar distribution of the *outcome* class (the obtained datasets are balanced).

3.4   Modeling

This phase consisted in exploring and choosing the ML models to use, always bearing in mind that this is a problem of classification. Therefore, taking into account [16], it was decided to apply five different ML techniques: **Logistic Regression** (LR), **Naive Bayes** (NB), **Random Forest** (RF), **Gradient Boosted Trees** (GBT), with a learning rate of 0.05, and **k-NN**, with $K = 10$.

In addition to choosing the models to be applied, the strategy for training and evaluating each of the selected ML models was also specified.

First, the dataset is split in two sub-datasets: 70% of dataset is used to train the ML model and the remaining 30% is used to test the obtained model. To train the ML model, it's used the Cross Validation technique with 50 folds and, then, after the training is completed, the ML model is tested with the testing dataset, obtaining the evaluation metrics. The number of folds to use in Cross Validation was chosen after some experimentation, and the selected value was the one that gave better overall results, without any evidence of over-fitting or under-fitting.

Figure 2 shows the implementation of the specified strategy, on RapidMiner.

3.5   Evaluation

Being the problem in hands a classification one, it was decided not to only use accuracy as performance metric, because it becomes misleading. Instead, it was used the combination of **F1 Score**, **Accuracy**, **Precision** and **Recall** to compare models, [17].

To clarify these concepts:

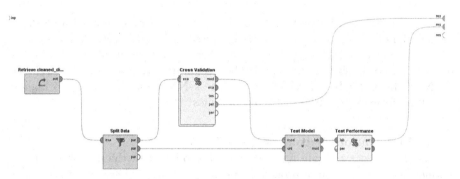

Fig. 2. Base modeling approach

- **Accuracy** - the ratio of correctly predicted examples to the total examples.
- **Precision** - the fraction of correctly classified positive examples from all classified as positive.
- **Recall** - actual positive rate of all positive examples, that is, the fraction of correctly classified examples.
- **F1 Score** - weighted average of Precision and Recall.

These concepts have mathematical representations, as follows:

- $Precision = \frac{TP}{TP+FP}$
- $Recall = \frac{TP}{TP+FN}$
- $F1Score = 2 * \frac{Recall*Precision}{Recall+Precision}$

Furthermore, the results presented next were calculated as the average of three different executions for each ML model.

(Data Preparation) First Approach
To begin with, the models were trained and tested with the dataset that resulted from the first data preparation approach. The Table 2 shows an overview of the results of each models for that dataset.

Table 2. ML model - testing results (1st approach)

ML model	Accuracy (%)	Precision (%)	Recall (%)	F1 score (%)
LR	78.55	79.35	77.63	78.38
NB	76.15	76.66	78.38	75.21
RF	93.51	94.09	93.62	93.76
GBT	96.60	96.62	96.61	96.55
k-NN	97.53	97.61	97.58	97.55

As it can be seen in Table 2, both the Logistic Regression and Naive Bayes model originated very low and unsatisfying results in every metric of evaluation, which is a clear indication that these models are not the most suitable to the prediction and classification at hand. The remaining three models: RF, GBT and k-NN produced far better results, being the k-NN model the one with highest overall performance with an F1 Score of almost 98%.

(Data Preparation) Second Approach
The next step was to train and test de ML models with the dataset from the second data preparation approach, given that the latter describes the problem more accurately. The Table 3 summarizes the obtained results for each ML model.

Table 3. ML model - testing results (2nd approach)

ML model	Accuracy (%)	Precision (%)	Recall (%)	F1 score (%)
LR	76.68	76.74	75.86	77.31
NB	73.32	73.32	73.33	73.51
RF	86.62	86.97	87.68	86.22
GBT	87.54	87.99	87.62	87.93
k-NN	89.94	90.35	90.08	90.17

As it was the case in the first dataset, the overall performance of the LR and NB was worst than the RF, GBT and k-NN models. Similarly, the k-NN model showed itself as the most suitable for the problem at hand, with an accuracy of 89%, precision and recall of 90% and, more importantly, with a F1 score of 90%.

4   Discussion

This section will address and discuss the overall strategies applied during the execution of the present work and, also, the achieved results.

In an early phase of data understanding it was clear that the used dataset was skewed, meaning that there was a bigger weight of instances on a class (in this case, the instances classified as NO), jeopardizing the applicability of ML models, which delivered a poorer predictive performance. Prior to the data preparation phase, there were some early experimentation with the already specified models which proved the previous thesis that the skewed data would produce weaker models and that it was an issue needed to be addressed.

Two datasets were produced with different approaches. The first approach was prepared in a way that the best results would be obtained when applying different models, but turned out to not be representative of the problem since the data was multiplied over and over again to balance the dataset and give the best possible performance. This resulted in ML models theoretically good (with good metrics in both training and testing, which was due to dataset having too much repeated examples) that had no real applicability in the problem. Because it was considered inadequate, although with good results, a second strategy was developed where the results did not perform as well as in the first approach but are more fit to the problem and, therefore, was considered as the final solution.

When modeling, five different models were chosen to be applied: LR, NB, RF, GBT and k-NN and the dataset was split into 70% for training and the remaining 30% for testing. To train the model a Cross Validation technique was used and after that, the model was tested. This methodology allows the processes to be more consistent and coherent between the multiple tests and execution, which provides more certainty regarding the ability to compare results and reproduce the described conditions in future iterations.

When evaluating the first approach, it was noticed that the overall performance metrics were acceptable when using RF, GBT and k-NN, because they had an F1 Score over 90%. LR and NB were not considered suitable since the achieved values were around 77%. Since k-NN obtained F1 Score values of 97%, it was considered the most valuable model for this approach.

In the final approach, NB and LR presented the worst performance with 77% and 73% of F1 Score, respectively. Improvement was seen on the other three models, with performances over 86%. RF and GBT had similar results but GBT had an overall improvement, having a F1 Score of 86% and 87%, respectively. With a F1 score of 90%, the k-NN model proved itself as the most suitable to the given problem and dataset.

Finally, although the results were not as good as in [11], the work in that paper was found difficult to replicate, even with the same dataset, primarily due to the low detail on the applied data preparation techniques, which leads to an even bigger difficulty of comparing results.

5   Conclusions and Future Work

This work had the purpose to build a model capable of predicting whether a person, more specifically, a women from the Pima Indian community, has diabetes or not. Given the dataset, acceptable results were achieved with the k-NN model with the second approach of data preparation with an overall performance of 90% of Accuracy, Precision, Recall and F1 Score.

The biggest obstacles to attain a successful model were mainly related to the dataset: it had much more instances of non-diabetes cases than diabetes ones and also had a large amount of missing values.

The work that is more prone to future improvement is: try to use a better oversampling technique to generate synthetic data instead of replicate the existent data, try a different overall approach to deal with the missing values and, finally, try other ML models of unsupervised learning.

Acknowledgements. This work is funded by "FCT-Fundação para a Cincia e Tecnologia" within the R&D Units Project Scope: UIDB/00319/2020.

References

1. Organization, W.H: Diabetes - Fact Sheet. https://www.who.int/en/news-room/fact-sheets/detail/diabetes. Accessed 05 June 2021
2. Aljumah, A.A., Ahamad, M.G., Siddiqui, M.K.: Application of data mining: diabetes health care in young and old patients. J. King Saud Univ. Comput. Inf. Sci. 25(2), 127–136 (2013). https://doi.org/10.1016/j.jksuci.2012.10.003, https://www.sciencedirect.com/science/article/pii/S1319157812000390
3. Witten, I.H., Frank, E., Hall, M.A.: Chapter 1 - what's it all about? In: Witten, I.H., Frank, E., Hall, M.A. (eds.) Data Mining: Practical Machine Learning Tools and Techniques, pp. 3–38. 3rd edn. The Morgan Kaufmann Series in Data Management Systems, Morgan Kaufmann, Boston (2011). https://doi.org/10.1016/B978-0-12-374856-0.00001-8, https://www.sciencedirect.com/science/article/pii/B9780123748560000018
4. Raghupathi, W., Raghupathi, V.: Big data analytics in healthcare: promise and potential. Health Inf. Sci. Syst. 2014 (2014)
5. Cruz, M., Esteves, M., Peixoto, H., Abelha, A., Machado, J.: Application of data mining for the prediction of prophylactic measures in patients at risk of deep vein thrombosis. In: Rocha, Á., Adeli, H., Reis, L.P., Costanzo, S. (eds.) New Knowledge in Information Systems and Technologies, pp. 557–567. Springer International Publishing, Cham (2019). https://doi.org/10.1007/978-3-030-16187-3_54
6. Konda, S., Rani, B., Govardhan, D.: Applications of data mining techniques in healthcare and prediction of heart attacks. Int. J. Comput. Sci. Eng. 2, 250–255 (2010)
7. Peixoto, H., et al.: Predicting postoperative complications for gastric cancer patients using data mining. In: Cortez, P., Magalhães, L., Branco, P., Portela, C.F., Adão, T. (eds.) Intelligent Technologies for Interactive Entertainment, pp. 37–46. Springer International Publishing, Cham (2019). https://doi.org/10.1007/978-3-030-16447-8_4
8. Loreto, P., Peixoto, H., Abelha, A., Machado, J.: Predicting low birth weight babies through data mining. In: Rocha, Á., Adeli, H., Reis, L.P., Costanzo, S. (eds.) New Knowledge in Information Systems and Technologies, pp. 568–577. Springer International Publishing, Cham (2019). https://doi.org/10.1007/978-3-030-16187-3_55
9. Silva, C., Oliveira, D., Peixoto, H., Machado, J., Abelha, A.: Data mining for prediction of length of stay of cardiovascular accident inpatients. In: Alexandrov, D.A., Boukhanovsky, A.V., Chugunov, A.V., Kabanov, Y., Koltsova, O. (eds.) Digital Transformation and Global Society, pp. 516–527. Springer International Publishing, Cham (2018). https://doi.org/10.1007/978-3-030-02843-5_43
10. Alpan, K., İlgi, G.S.: Classification of diabetes dataset with data mining techniques by using weka approach. In: 2020 4th International Symposium on Multidisciplinary Studies and Innovative Technologies (ISMSIT), pp. 1–7 (2020). https://doi.org/10.1109/ISMSIT50672.2020.9254720
11. Wu, H., Yang, S., Huang, Z., He, J., Wang, X.: Type 2 diabetes mellitus prediction model based on data mining. Inf. Med. Unlock. 10, 100–107 (2018). https://doi.org/10.1016/j.imu.2017.12.006, https://www.sciencedirect.com/science/article/pii/S2352914817301405

12. Portela, F., Santos, M.F., Machado, J., Abelha, A., Rua, F., Silva, Á.: Real-time decision support using data mining to predict blood pressure critical events in intensive medicine patients. In: Bravo, J., Hervás, R., Villarreal, V. (eds.) Ambient Intelligence for Health, pp. 77–90. Springer International Publishing, Cham (2015). https://doi.org/10.1007/978-3-319-26508-7_8

13. Guide, I.S.M.C.D: ftp://ftp.software.ibm.com/software/analytics/spss/document ation/modeler/14.2/en.CRISP_DM.pdf (2011)

14. Witten, I.H., Frank, E.: Data mining: practical machine learning tools and techniques with java implementations. ACM SIGMOD Rec. **31**(1), 76–77 (2002)

15. Wirth, R., Hipp, J.: Crisp-dm: towards a standard process model for data mining. In: Proceedings of the 4th International Conference on the Practical Applications of Knowledge Discovery and Data Mining (2000)

16. Wu, X., Kumar, V., Quinlan, J.R., Ghosh, J., Yang, Q., Motoda, H., McLachlan, G.J., Ng, A., Liu, B., Philip, S.Y., et al.: Top 10 algorithms in data mining. Knowl. Inf. Syst. **14**(1), 1–37 (2008)

17. Hossin, M., Sulaiman, M.N.: A review on evaluation metrics for data classification evaluations. Int. J. Data Mining Knowl. Manage. Process **5**(2), 01–11 (2015). https://doi.org/10.5121/ijdkp.2015.5201

Not Just a Matter of Accuracy: A fNIRS Pilot Study into Discrepancy Between Sleep Data and Subjective Sleep Experience in Quantified-Self Sleep Tracking

Zilu Liang[1,2(✉)] [iD]

[1] Ubiquitous Computing and Personal Informatics Lab, Kyoto University of Advanced Science (KUAS), Kyoto, Japan
liang.zilu@kuas.ac.jp
[2] Institute of Industrial Science (IIS), The University of Tokyo, Tokyo, Japan

Abstract. Quantified-self sleep tracking devices such as Fitbit are gaining great popular in recent years. However, users often complain about the discrepancy between the data collected with sleep trackers and their subjective sleep experience, which is often attributed to the accuracy issue of the devices. In this pilot study, we aim to provide an explanation to such discrepancy from a neuroscience perspective. We investigated the associations of subjective sleep rating and Fitbit measured sleep data to cortical hemodynamics in the prefrontal cortex (PFC) during the first sleep cycle. Correlation analysis results showed that subjective sleep rating mainly correlated to the median of the concentration changes in oxyhemoglobin ($\Delta O2Hb$) and deoxyhemoglobin (ΔHHb) in a set of channels, with positive correlation coefficients. In contrast, the sleep score computed by Fitbit mainly correlated to the mean of the $\Delta O2Hb$ and ΔHHb in a different set of channels, with negative correlation coefficients. The findings suggested that better perceived sleep quality may be positively associated to increased hemodynamics during the first sleep cycle, and the opposite may be true for objective sleep metrics such as sleep score measured by Fitbit. The result implies that users' subjective perception of sleep and the sleep tracking devices may be capturing different dimensions of sleep. As such, improving device accuracy may help little in addressing the discrepancy between the subjective sleep experience and the objective data. The findings provided design implications for the development of future sleep tracking technologies.

Keywords: Quantified-Self · Sleep tracking · Fitbit · fNIRS

1 Introduction

Sleep health has far-reaching effects on people's mental and physical health [1]. The past decade has witnessed significantly advances in quantified-self sleep tracking technologies that allow users to monitor their sleep at home and over an extended time

S. Spinsante et al. (Eds.): HealthyIoT 2021, LNICST 432, pp. 74–87, 2022.
https://doi.org/10.1007/978-3-030-99197-5_7

span. Popular devices like Fitbit and Apple Watch allow users to measure clinically significant sleep variables with reasonable accuracy [2, 3], and have been increasingly used in research studies to measure sleep outcomes for better ecological validity [4–6]. These devices use embedded accelerometer and photoplethysmogram (PPG) to infer the sleep stages that a user goes through at night. Many studies have investigated how users interact with sleep tracking technologies in various forms (e.g., wristbands, headbands, smartphone apps) [4, 7–9], and found that users often complained about the discrepancy between the data collected with these devices and their subjective sleep experience [7, 8]. Such discrepancy also often causes cognitive dissonance that reduces users' trust of the devices and drive them to discontinue their use [7].

The discrepancy between the data measured with sleep trackers and users' subjective sleep experience is often referred to as an accuracy issue, which leads researchers to assume that improving device accuracy is the solution to the problem. Nonetheless, sleep science studies found that the discrepancy between the sleep data and the subjective sleep experience may persist even when the gold standard sleep measurement technique— polysomnography (PSG)—is used, suggesting that such discrepancy is likely to be less a matter of device accuracy but rather a common phenomenon in human sleep. Prior sleep research studies show that sleep metrics derived from PSG data explained poorly the variance in subjective sleep quality [10, 11]. A recent study on how users interact with sleep tracking technology argues that there is no one-on-one mapping between the objective sleep metrics and the subjective sleep quality, despite that users tend to establish a false connection between their subjective sleep experience and some sleep metrics [7]. For example, sleep metrics such as micro-arousals, deep sleep, and REM sleep can barely be consciously perceived, but users tend to use them as a proxy of their subjective sleep quality.

Despite the commonplace of the discrepancy between the objective sleep data and the subjective sleep experience, the mechanism of this phenomenon is poorly understood especially in the domain of the quantified-self sleep tracking. In this pilot study, we sought to provide an explanation to the discrepancy between quantified-self sleep data recorded with Fitbit and subjective sleep experience from a neuroscience perspective. We investigated the associations of the subjective sleep rating and the Fitbit measured sleep data to cortical hemodynamics in the prefrontal cortex (PFC) during the first sleep cycle. This study is the first attempt to bring a neuroscience perspective to the study of quantified-self sleep tracking. The preliminary results implied that the device measured sleep data and subjective sleep experience may characterize different aspects of the sleep process, indicating that the discrepancy between the two may not be easily addressed by simply improving device accuracy. We pointed out directions for future sleep tracking research based on our findings.

2 Related Work

Advances in wearable and mobile computing technologies have witnessed a sharp increase in the adoption of quantified-self sleep tracking technologies in recent years. These sleep tracking technologies largely fall into two categories. The first category supports users to manually log subjective sleep experience either using validated psychometric questionnaires (e.g., the Pittsburgh Sleep Quality Index; PSQI [12]) or a simple

Likert rating scale. These technologies are often made available to users in the form of a stand-alone mobile app, or as one feature in a comprehensive sleep tracking system (e.g., SleepAsAndroid, SleepBot). The other category leverages wearable or mobile sensors to objectively measure a user's sleep structure. These technologies often require users to put on a wearable tracker or to place a smartphone on bed. Popular trackers include Fitbit, Apple Watch, Mi Band and Oura Ring. Using proprietary algorithms, these devices approximate sleep structure metrics including total sleep time (TST), wake after sleep onset (WASO), sleep efficiency (SE), and sleep stages. Different devices may also have self-defined sleep metrics such as the sleep score by Fitbit, which is a weighted sum of several sleep metrics.

Studies of quantified-self sleep tracking technologies have dominantly focused on their validity/accuracy and usability. Despite of their convenience for longitudinal use in daily life settings, quantified-self sleep tracking devices may have limited accuracy depending on the type of sensors used [9]. The validity of popular sleep trackers has been well-studied in both laboratories [13] and naturalistic settings [2]. Recent findings showed that the latest models achieved reasonable accuracy for TST and SE, but not for sleep stages [2, 13]. In addition, device accuracy was found to correlate to many factors including the demographic characteristics and the sleep structure of the users [3, 21], and may also demonstrate temporal patterns [20]. The usability of quantified-self sleep trackers was also intensively studied. Previous studies have investigated how users interpret sleep data [4], users' trust towards sleep tracking technologies [7], and the challenges for these technologies to improve sleep health [9].

A common complaint related to quantified-self sleep tracking technologies is the mismatch between sleep data and users' subjective sleep experience [7]. Such mismatch is often attributed to the limited accuracy of the sleep trackers, and it is believed that improving device accuracy could help bridge the gap between the two. Nonetheless, the discrepancy between objective sleep data and subjective sleep quality has been observed even when the gold standard of sleep measurement—polysomnography (PSG)—was used. Several medical studies have demonstrated that PSG did not explain subjective sleep quality well [10]. The sleep structural metrics measured with PSG explained only 11–17% of the variance in subjective sleep quality. Discrepancy between device measured sleep structure and perceived sleep quality has been observed not only in patients with Alzheimer disease, depression, and sleep problems, but also in healthy adults [14]. For example, one study shows that healthy people who habitually slept more than 6 h at night may both overestimate and underestimate their sleep duration. In addition, the rate of overestimation significantly increased by 3 times among healthy people who slept less than 6 h at night [15]. A recent usability study into how users perceive the credibility of consumer sleep trackers also found that even when these sleep trackers agreed well to a medical reference, they not necessarily match the users' subjective sleep experience [7].

In this study, we attempted to approach the sleep misperception phenomenon from a neuroscience perspective within the context of quantified-self sleep tracking. We investigated the associations of subjective sleep rating and Fitbit measured sleep data to cortical hemodynamics in the prefrontal cortex (PFC) during the first sleep cycle. While we solely focused on Fitbit as a representative of quantified-self sleep tracking technologies, the methodology adopted in this study is readily applicable to sleep trackers of other manufacturers. This study generated new insights into the discrepancy between consumer device measured sleep data and subjective sleep experience and pointed out directions for future sleep tracking research.

3 Measuring Devices and Instruments

3.1 Wearable fNIRS System

In this study, we measured the cortical hemodynamics using a wearable functional near-infrared spectroscopy (fNIRS): the Brite 24 system developed by the Artinits Medical System Co., The Netherland. The Brite 24 measures the concentration changes of the oxyhemoglobin ($\Delta O2Hb$) and deoxyhemoglobin (ΔHHb) in cortical brain areas. Compared to other hemodynamic imaging methods such as fMRI and PET, fNIRS is less invasive, more tolerant to motion artefacts, and allows higher temporal resolution. Compared to EEG, fNIRS has the advantage of higher spatial resolution.

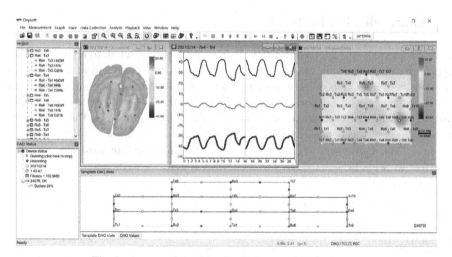

Fig. 1. A screenshot of the OxySoft companion software.

While traditional fNIRS systems often involves using bulky devices and many long cables, the Brite 24 system is a wearable and ready-to-use device that requires little set up time. The system contains 10 transmitters (Tx) that emit infrared light at the wavelengths of 760 nm and 850 nm. The infrared light travels through the sculp, the skull and the cortex. The rebounded light is captured by 8 receivers (Rx). Using the template as shown in the bottom of Fig. 1, the Txs and Rxs were configured into 27 channels, with an interoptode distance of 3 cm and penetration depth of 1.5 cm. The optodes were fixed on a soft neoprene head cap and were placed between the FpZ-F3-Cz-F4-FpZ region according to the international 10–20 EEG system. Using the neoprene head cap not only makes it easy to install and uninstall the optodes, but also ensure that the optodes were placed in the same location across different measurements. The fNIRS system has a companion software called OxySoft (Artinits Medical System Co., The Netherland). All the measurements in this study were conducted online, where the Brite 24 device was connected to the OxySoft via Bluetooth. In this way, data were regularly synchronized with the OxySoft. A screenshot of the OxySoft is illustrated in Fig. 1.

3.2 Fitbit Sense and Sleep Rating

We used Fitbit Sense—the latest model of Fitbit at the time of the study—to measure a set of sleep metrics. These metrics include total sleep time (TST), wake after sleep onset (WASO), wake ratio (WR), light sleep ratio (LR), deep sleep ratio (DR), REM sleep ratio (RR), and sleep score (SS). Participants worn the device on their non-dominant wrist and the data were automatically collected without requiring any manual input. Sleep data were synchronized with the Fitbit smartphone app the next morning upon waking up. Subjective sleep quality was collected using a 1–5 Likert scale, with 1 and 5 denoting extremely poor sleep and extremely good sleep, respectively.

4 Data Collection Protocol

In this pilot study, we adopted the N-of-1 single subject research design [16, 17]. This approach differs from the traditional cross-sectional study design in that it does not rely on the assumption of cohort homogeneity. We collected data from one healthy male participant who is Caucasian and was in his 30s. The participant did not have any diagnosed health conditions, mental problems, or sleep problems. The data collection experiment was conducted at the participant's home following a protocol listed in Table 1. The participant volunteered to shave his hair to minimize any potential interference with the signal quality of the fNIRS system.

Table 1. Data collection protocol.

Event ID	Time	Event	Device and Instrument
1	Between 22:30–23:30	Rest quietly while staying awake for 2 min	Brite 24, Fitbit Sense
2	Right after Event 1	Get in bed and lights off	Brite 24, Fitbit Sense
3	The first major wake	Take off Brite 24 and stop the measurement	/
4	Upon waking up 6:30–7:30	Rate subjective sleep quality	A 1–5 Likert scale

5 Data Analysis Protocol

The raw optical density (OD) signals recorded with Brite 24 were exported into EDF files using the companion software OxySoft. The EDF files were converted to fNIRS data type and then processed using the MNE-NIRS Python library. The OD signals of each night were trimmed between sleep start time T_S (as recorded by the Fitbit Sense) and $T_S + 90$ min, which is the average length of a sleep cycle in healthy adults. The OD signal quality of each channel was analyzed using the scalp coupling index (SCI) method [18]. For each channel, the OD signals at both wavelengths were passed through a bandpass filter (0.7–1.5 Hz) to preserve only the heartbeat component. The SCI—defined as the zero-lag cross-correlation between the heartbeat component of the OD signals at both wavelengths—was then calculated and used as an indicator of the signal quality of the channel. Channels with an SCI below 0.75 were discarded. The processed OD signals were converted to ΔO2Hb and ΔHHb using the modified Beer-Lambert law (MBLL) [19], and bandpass filtered (0.02–0.18 Hz) to remove the cardiac and respiratory noise. Five time-domain features (i.e., mean, median, standard deviation, skewness, kurtosis) and three frequency-domain features (i.e., total power, peak amplitude of the frequency components, peak ratio) were derived from the ΔO2Hb and ΔHHb signals of each channel and then averaged across all channels.

Table 2. List of variables used in correlation analysis.

Category	Metric (Denotation)	Data type	Device and instrument
Cortical ΔO2Hb and ΔHHb	Mean (*mean_O2*/*mean_H*)	Continuous	Brite 24
	Median (*md_O2*/*md_H*)		
	Standard deviation (*sd_O2*/*sd_H*)		
	Skewness (*sk_O2*/*sk_H*)		
	Kurtosis (*kt_O2*/*kt_H*)		
	Total power (*tp_O2*/*tp_H*)		
	Maximum power (*mf_O2*/*mf_H*)		
	Peak ratio (*pr_O2*/*pr_H*)		
Sleep	Sleep rating (*SR*)	Ordinal	A 1–5 Likert scale
	Sleep score (*SS*)	Continuous	Fitbit sense
	Total sleep time (*TST*)		
	Wake after sleep onset (*WASO*)		
	Wake ratio (*WR*)		
	Light sleep ratio (*LR*)		
	Deep sleep ratio (*DR*)		
	REM sleep ratio (*RR*)		

The Fitbit sleep data were exported using a web application that we developed in our previous study [4]. These data were then merged with the participant's subjective sleep rating and the features derived from the hemodynamic signals by matching the date stamps. Table 2 summarizes the metrics that were used in the correlation analysis. Pearson's and Spearman's correlation coefficients were calculated pair-wisely on continuous metrics and ordinal metrics, separately. Statistical test at a significance level of $\alpha = 0.05$ was performed. Correlation coefficients were calculated using the Pandas library and statistical test was performed using the SciPy library in Python 3.8.

6 Results

The significant correlations between sleep metrics (both sleep rating and Fitbit measured sleep data) and hemodynamic features are shown in Table 3. It shows that subjective sleep rating was moderately and negatively correlated to the average sk and kt of the $\Delta O2Hb$. No significant correlation was found between the subjective sleep rating and the features derived from ΔHHb.

Table 3. Statistically significant correlations between sleep metrics and average hemodynamic features.

Sleep metric	Feature	r	p	Sleep metric	Feature	r	p
SR	sk_O2	−0.516	0.049	TST	md_O2	−0.648	0.016
	kt_O2	−0.516	0.049		mf_O2	0.603	0.029
SS	sd_O2	−0.717	0.006		md_H	−0.59	0.034
	sd_H	−0.731	0.005	DR	sd_O2	−0.611	0.026
	sk_H	−0.589	0.034		sd_H	−0.594	0.032
	kt_H	−0.59	0.034		sk_H	−0.554	0.049
RR	sk_O2	−0.692	0.009	WR	mean_O2	0.735	0.004
	kt_O2	−0.716	0.006	LR	sd_O2	0.730	0.005
	tp_O2	0.673	0.012		sk_O2	0.726	0.005
	mf_O2	−0.653	0.015		kt_O2	0.698	0.008
	pr_O2	0.687	0.009		tp_O2	−0.538	0.058
	sd_H	−0.568	0.043		pr_O2	−0.599	0.031
	sk_H	−0.614	0.025		sd_H	0.728	0.005
	kt_H	−0.640	0.018		sk_H	0.745	0.003
	tp_H	0.663	0.013		kt_H	0.751	0.003
	mf_H	−0.695	0.008		pr_H	−0.702	0.007
	pr_H	0.728	0.005				

Table 4. Statistically significant correlations between subjective sleep rating and channel-wise hemodynamic features.

Rx-Tx pair	Feature	r	p
Rx3_Tx2	*md_O2*	0.514	0.050
	md_H	−0.633	0.011
Rx4_Tx3	*md_H*	0.571	0.026
	sk_H	0.561	0.030
Rx4_Tx4	*md_O2*	−0.573	0.025
	md_H	−0.531	0.042
	sk_H	0.514	0.050
Rx4_Tx5	*sk_O2*	0.691	0.004
	md_H	−0.599	0.018
Rx4_Tx8	*md_O2*	0.548	0.034
Rx5_Tx7	*sk_H*	0.620	0.014
Rx6_Tx8	*md_O2*	0.665	0.007
Rx7_Tx10	*md_O2*	0.629	0.012

Table 5. Statistically significant correlations between Fitbit sleep score and channel-wise hemodynamic features.

Rx-Tx pair	Feature	r	p
Rx2_Tx3	*mean_H*	−0.805	<0.001
Rx2_Tx4	*mean_O2*	−0.670	0.012
	mean_H	−0.594	0.032
	md_H	−0.611	0.026
Rx3_Tx2	*mean_H*	−0.639	0.019
	md_H	−0.664	0.033
Rx3_Tx3	*mean_O2*	−0.599	0.030
	mean_H	−0.777	0.023
Rx3_Tx5	*mean_O2*	−0.852	0.007
Rx4_Tx5	*mean_H*	−0.703	0.007
Rx4_Tx8	*mean_H*	0.998	0.043
Rx5_Tx5	*mean_O2*	−0.999	0.033
Rx6_Tx9	*mean_H*	−0.740	0.023
Rx7_Tx7	*mean_H*	−0.717	0.006
Rx7_Tx8	*mean_O2*	−0.571	0.041
Rx8_Tx8	*mean_O2*	−0.926	0.003

Different objective sleep metrics as measured with Fitbit Sense correlated to different hemodynamic features. Strong correlations ($|r| > 0.700$) were found between sleep score and the sd of $\Delta O2Hb$ and ΔHHb, wake ratio and the *mean* of $\Delta O2Hb$, light sleep ratio and the sd, sk of $\Delta O2Hb$ and the sd, sk, kt, pr of ΔHHb, REM sleep ratio and the kt of $\Delta O2Hb$ and the pr of ΔHHb.

Table 4 and 5 show the statistically significant correlations between channel-wise hemodynamic features and subjective sleep rating, sleep score computed by Fitbit, respectively. Figure 2 shows a coarse visualization of the channel-wise correlations. Strong positive and negative correlation are indicated by red and dark blue connections. Moderate positive and negative correlations are indicated by orange and light blue. Grey double lines indicate both positive and negative correlations were observed. It is observed that the subjective sleep rating mainly correlated to the median of the $\Delta O2Hb$ and ΔHHb in certain channels, with positive correlation coefficients. In contrast, the sleep score computed by Fitbit mainly correlates to the mean the $\Delta O2Hb$ and ΔHHb in a different set of channels, with negative correlation coefficients.

Table 6 shows the statistically significant correlations between channel-wise hemodynamic features and other Fitbit measured sleep metrics. Figure 3, 4, 5 shows a coarse visualization of the corresponding channel-wise correlations. Broken down into sleep metrics that characterize different dimensions of the sleep structure, the total sleep time and deep sleep were mostly negatively correlated to the PFC hemodynamics, while sleep efficiency, wake after sleep onset, wake ratio and light sleep ratio (note that these features all characterize the continuity of sleep) were mostly positively correlated to the PFC hemodynamics. No correlation was observed between REM sleep ratio and the channel-wise hemodynamic features.

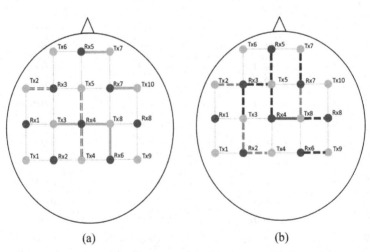

(a)   (b)

Fig. 2. A visualization of the channel-wise correlations between (a) the subjective sleep rating and the hemodynamic features, and (b) the Fitbit sleep score and the hemodynamic features. Strong positive and negative correlation are indicated by red and dark blue connections. Moderate positive and negative correlations are indicated by orange and light blue connections. Grey double lines indicate both positive and negative correlations were observed. (Color figure online)

Table 6. Statistically significant correlations between Fitbit measured sleep metrics and channel-wise hemodynamic features.

Sleep metrics	Rx-Tx pair	Feature	r	p
TST	Rx2_Tx3	*mean_H*	−0.573	0.041
	Rx2_Tx4	*md_H*	−0.586	0.035
	Rx3_Tx3	*mean_O2*	−0.599	0.030
		mean_H	−0.842	0.009
	Rx3_Tx5	*mean_O2*	−0.797	0.018
	Rx6_Tx9	*mean_H*	−0.694	0.038
	Rx8_Tx8	*mean_O2*	−0.853	0.015
WASO	Rx3_Tx2	*sk_O2*	0.705	0.005
		kt_O2	−0.751	0.002
	Rx5_Tx7	*sk_O2*	0.844	<0.001
SE	Rx8_Tx10	*pr_O2*	0.642	0.018
WR	Rx2_Tx3	*mean_H*	0.677	0.011
	Rx5_Tx5	*mean_H*	0.999	0.019
LR	Rx2_Tx4	*mean_O2*	0.581	0.037
		mean_H	0.573	0.041
	Rx3_Tx2	*mean_H*	0.569	0.042
	Rx3_Tx5	*mean_O2*	0.719	0.045
	Rx6_Tx9	*mean_O2*	0.611	0.046
	Rx7_Tx8	*mean_O2*	0.566	0.044
		mean_H	0.566	0.044
	Rx8_Tx8	*mean_O2*	0.801	0.030
	Rx6_Tx4	*sk_H*	0.556	0.049
DR	Rx2_Tx4	*mean_H*	−0.641	0.018
	Rx3_Tx2	*mean_H*	−0.660	0.014
	Rx3_Tx5	*mean_O2*	−0.781	0.022
	Rx4_Tx5	*mean_H*	−0.568	0.043
		md_H	−0.572	0.041
	Rx5_Tx5	*mean_H*	−0.999	0.019
	Rx7_Tx7	*mean_H*	−0.616	0.025
	Rx7_Tx8	*mean_O2*	−0.624	0.023
		mean_H	−0.553	0.050
	Rx8_Tx8	*mean_O2*	−0.783	0.037

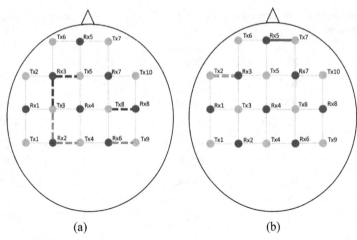

Fig. 3. A visualization of the channel-wise correlations between (a) total sleep time and hemodynamic features, and (b) wake after sleep onset and hemodynamic features.

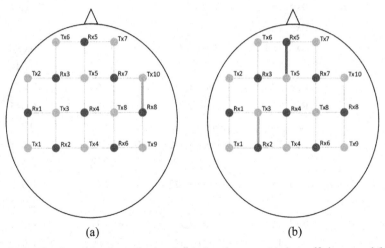

Fig. 4. A visualization of the channel-wise correlations between (a) sleep efficiency, and (b) wake ratio and hemodynamic features.

7   Discussions

The correlation analysis results show that subjective sleep rating was moderately and negatively correlated to the average skewness and kurtosis of the ΔO2Hb, but not significantly correlated to features derived from ΔHHb. Different objective sleep metrics as measured with Fitbit correlate to different hemodynamic features. Channel-wisely, it is found that subjective sleep rating mainly correlates to the median of the ΔO2Hb and ΔHHb in a set of channels, with positive correlation coefficients. In contrast, the sleep score computed by Fitbit mainly correlates to the mean the ΔO2Hb and ΔHHb in a different set of channels, with negative correlation coefficients. This suggests that better perceived sleep quality may be positively associated to increased hemodynamics during the first sleep cycle, and the opposite is true for objective sleep metrics as measured by Fitbit. Sleep metrics related to the continuity of sleep—including WASO, SE, WR—and LR were positively associated to increased hemodynamics in the PFC during the first sleep cycle, while sleep metrics such as TST and DR were negatively associated to increased hemodynamics in the PFC during the first sleep cycle.

The analysis results imply that the discrepancy between subjective sleep experience and objective sleep data is likely due to the mismatch of the measurands. Since users' subjective consciousness and the sleep tracking device are essentially measuring different dimensions of sleep, it is reasonable to expect certain level of discrepancy between the two. As such, improving device accuracy may not help solve the discrepancy. Instead, designing future sleep tracking technologies that help users to understand the sleep misperception phenomenon could be a more plausible direction to go. It would also be interesting to explore the objective sleep metrics that correlate well to each user's subjective sleep rating, and to use them as personalized indicators of sleep quality rather than using a general set of metrics for all users like the current technologies do.

Due to the N-of-1 approach adopted in this study, the findings solely hold for this specific subject. In our future study, we plan to repeat the study protocol with a cohort of subjects to identify potential common patterns across subjects.

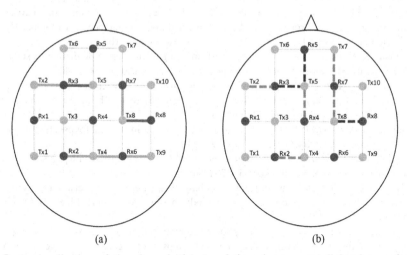

(a)   (b)

Fig. 5. A visualization of the channel-wise correlations between (a) light sleep ratio and hemodynamic features, and (b) deep sleep ratio and hemodynamic features.

Acknowledgement. This work was supported by the Japan Society for the Promotion of Science (JSPS) KAKENHI Grant Number 16H07469, 19K20141, and 21K17670.

References

1. Buysse, D.J.: Sleep health: can we define it? does it matter? Sleep **37**(1), 9–17 (2014)
2. Liang, Z., Chapa-Martell, M.A.: Validity of consumer activity wristbands and wearable EEG for measuring overall sleep parameters and sleep structure in free-living conditions. J. Healthcare Inf. Res. **2**(1–2), 152–178 (2018)
3. Liang, Z., Chapa-Martell, M.A.: Accuracy of Fitbit wristbands in measuring sleep stage transitions and the effect of user-specific factors. JMIR Mhealth Uhealth **7**(6), e13384 (2019)
4. Liang, Z., et al.: SleepExplorer: a visualization tool to make sense of correlations between personal sleep data and contextual factors. Pers. Ubiquit. Comput. **20**(6), 985–1000 (2016). https://doi.org/10.1007/s00779-016-0960-6
5. Weatherall, J., et al.: Sleep tracking and exercise in patients with type 2 diabetes mellitus (step-D): pilot study to determine correlations between Fitbit data and patient-reported outcomes. JMIR Mhealth Uhealth **6**(6), e131 (2018)
6. Bian, J., et al.: Exploring the association between self-reported asthma impact and Fitbit-derived sleep quality and physical activity measures in adolescents. JMIR mHealth and uHealth **5**(7), e105 (2017)
7. Liang, Z., Ploderer, B.: How does Fitbit measure brainwaves: a qualitative study into the credibility of sleep-tracking technologies. Proc. ACM Interact. Mob. Wearable Ubiquitous Technol. **4**(1), Article 17 (2020)
8. Liu, W., Ploderer, B., Hoang, T.: In bed with technology: challenges and opportunities for sleep tracking. In: Proceedings of the Annual Meeting of the Australian Special Interest Group for Computer Human Interaction, pp. 142–151. Parkville, VIC, Australia (2015)
9. Liang, Z., Ploderer, B.: Sleep tracking in the real world: a qualitative study into barriers for improving sleep. In: Proceedings of the 28th Australian Conference on Computer-Human Interaction, pp. 537–541. Launceston, Tasmania, Australia (2016)
10. Kaplan, K.A., et al.: When a gold standard isn't so golden: lack of prediction of subjective sleep quality from sleep polysomnography. Biol. Psychol. **123**, 37–46 (2017)
11. Baker, F.C., Maloney, S., Driver, H.S.: A comparison of subjective estimates of subjective estimates of sleep with objective polysomnographic data in healthy men and women. J. Psychosom. Res. **47**(4), 335–341 (1999)
12. Buysse, D., et al.: The Pittsburgh sleep quality index: a new instrument for psychiatric practice and research. Psychiatry Res. **28**(2), 193–213 (1989)
13. De Zambotti, M., et al.: A validation study of Fitbit Charge 2 compared with polysomnography in adults. Chronobiol. Int. **35**(4), 465–476 (2017)
14. Hsiao, F.-C., et al.: The neurophysiological basis of the discrepancy between objective and subjective sleep during the sleep onset period: an EEG-fMRI study. Sleep **41**(6), zsy056 (2018)
15. Fernandez-Mendoza, J., et al.: Sleep misperception and chronic insomnia in the general population: the role of objective sleep duration and psychological profiles. Psychosom. Med. **73**(1), 88–97 (2011)
16. De Groot, M., et al.: Single subject (N-of-1) research design, data processing, and personal science. Methods Inf. Med. **6** (2017)
17. Shaffer, J.A., et al.: N-of-1 randomized intervention trials in health psychology: a systematic review and methodology critique. Ann. Behav. Med. **52**, 731–742 (2018)
18. Pollonini, L., et al.: Auditory cortex activation to natural speech and simulated cochlear implant speech measured with functional near-infrared spectroscopy. Hear. Res. **309**, 84–93 (2014)
19. Delpy, D.T., et al.: Estimation of optical pathlength through tissue from direct time of flight measurement. Phys. Med. Biol. **33**, 1433–1442 (1988)

20. Liang, Z., Chapa-Martell, M.A.: Combining numerical and visual approaches in validating sleep data quality of consumer wearable wristbands. In: Proceedings of IEEE PerCom Workshops (IQ2S Workshop), pp.777–782. Kyoto, Japan (2019)
21. Liang, Z., Chapa-Martell, M.A.: A multi-level classification approach for sleep stage prediction with processed data derived from consumer wearable activity trackers. Front. Dig. Health **3**, 665946 (2021)

Detection of Diabetic Retinopathy Using CNN

Raghad Abdulghani[(⊠)], Ghaida Albakri, Rawan Alraddadi, and Liyakathunisa Syed

College of Computer Science and Engineering, Taibah University, Madinah, Saudi Arabia
`raghad.at@gmail.com, {tu4160060,tu4160057}@taibahu.edu.sa,`
`lansari@taiabhu.edu.sa`

Abstract. Diabetic retinopathy is one of the most common diseases for diabetic patients around the world. Moreover, this disease causes lesions on the retina which affect the vision of the patient. Hence, diabetic retinopathy may lead to blindness in some cases if not detected earlier. Therefore, early detection of this disease is required to prevent vision loss. In this paper, deep learning techniques were used to produce a good performance in detecting and classifying fundus images. The proposed method is an implementation of CNN algorithm that detects and classifies fundus images based on the stage of the disease. As a result, the accuracy we obtained in our approach has reached 92.26% and MSE of 0.0628.

Keywords: CNN · Deep learning · Diabetic retinopathy · Median filter · Morphology · Interpolation

1 Introduction

Diabetes is a serious chronic disease that affects the lives of individuals, their families and society. It does not only affect adults, but children likewise. Moreover, it may occur in three situations: when the pancreas does not produce insulin, does not produce it properly or when the body cannot use the insulin produced by the pancreas [1]. Additionally, insulin is a hormone that allows glucose absorbed from food to pass from the blood flow into the cells to produce energy. According to the International Diabetes Federation, 463 million people around the world are diabetics. Moreover, 55 million of them are in the MENA region, 33.8 million in North America, 59 million are in Europe and 87.6 million are in the South East of Asia [1].

There are three types of diabetes: Type 1 Diabetes (T1D), Type 2 Diabetes (T2D) and Gestational Diabetes Mellitus (GDM) [2]. The first one occurs when the pancreas produces little to no insulin. Consequently, the patient needs a daily insulin injection to control the glucose level in the blood. As for the second, it occurs when the body does not use the insulin produced by the pancreas. Thus, it has various treatments such as: healthy lifestyle, oral drugs and insulin injection. Whereas, the third occurs during pregnancy when the mother has high level of glucose in her blood. Also, this type affects both the mother and the child. Even though glucose level decreases back to normal after pregnancy, some cases have shown that it evolves into type 2 diabetes [1].

S. Spinsante et al. (Eds.): HealthyIoT 2021, LNICST 432, pp. 88–98, 2022.
https://doi.org/10.1007/978-3-030-99197-5_8

Diabetic retinopathy is one of the complications of diabetes that requires an annual examination for early detection. Whereas, it occurs in type 1 and type 2 diabetes and is the most recurrent cause for blindness among adults [3]. As a definition, diabetic retinopathy is a diabetes complication that damages the blood vessels inside the retina causing blood and fluid leakage. Additionally, this leakage creates microaneurysms, exudates and hemorrhages [4]. Figure 1 shows how microaneurysms, exudates and hemorrhages look inside the eye using fundus photography [5]. Whereas, microaneurysms appear as small red dots inside blood vessels, exudates appear as yellow spots on the retina and hemorrhages appears as red spots which are usually larger than microaneurysms.

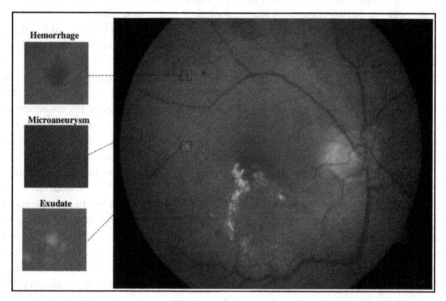

Fig. 1. Exudates, hemorrhages and microaneurysms inside the eye tissue [6].

The process of extracting retina blood vessels to determine the diseases is a time-consuming process. Therefore, automating the extraction process will help simplifying and accelerate the process. Also, detecting the diseases early will decrease the blindness risk by 95% [6, 7]. Hence, the proposed system aims to identify diabetic retinopathy using image processing and deep learning techniques. Thus, fundus photography images of the retina with different cases of diabetic retinopathy were used as a dataset [8]. As for the deep learning technique, Convolutional Neural Network (CNN) was used to classify the stage of the disease. Further, the four stages used for classification are: not detected, low, mild and severe.

The rest of the paper is organized as follows. Section 2 provides a background about the diabetic retinopathy disease and some basic information about deep learning, image processing and how they are combined. In Sect. 3, we provided some literature review on the previous image processing techniques that have been proposed by different researchers. In Sect. 4, we proposed the methodology we used to develop our method.

Section 5 discusses the results that we obtained. Whereas Sect. 6 provides the conclusion of our paper.

2 Background

2.1 Diabetic Retinopathy

One of the senses our body has is our eyes. They allow us to see and differentiate everything around us. Specifically, the light gets into the pupil-along with the iris and cornea's help-upon the retina. Then, the retina helps to convert the image so the brain can process the environment with the help of rods and cones. Thus, a healthy retina plays an important role in human vision. However, the retina can be affected by many diseases leading to blindness. Diabetic eye disease is the most common retina disease which includes: Diabetic Retinopathy, Glaucoma, and Cataract [9].

Diabetic Retinopathy is an eye disease that affects diabetic patients. In addition, it is considered to be the most popular one and it is the cause of visual weakness for adults. However, it is a consequence of an alteration in the retina blood vessels. In consequence, the retina is located in the eye rear and is described as the sensitive tissue. Moreover, the retina blood vessels in some cases of diabetic retinopathy tend to swell and leak fluid, while the growth of new blood vessels on the retina surface is the abnormal case.

Proliferative Diabetic Retinopathy (P.D.R) and Non-Proliferative Diabetic Retinopathy (NPDR) are the two stages of diabetic retinopathy [10]. NPDR is considered to be the early stage of diabetic retinopathy. Whereas, it happens when the blood vessels in the retina start to leak blood and fluids. Sometimes, these blood vessels might close off, causing what is called exudates. PDR on the other hand, is a more advanced and serious stage. Consequently, it occurs when new blood vessels start to grow. Accordingly, these blood vessels are fragile, so they bleed through the retina. If the vessels bleed a little, it causes dark floaters. And if they bleed a lot, it blocks the vision causing blindness [10].

2.2 Deep Learning Techniques

Deep learning methods have a huge impact on different fields, especially on medical image analysis which is considered a huge research area that has been developed in the last decade and is still improving. The reason for that is it helps us not only to identify the different diseases found by images, but it helps also to construct new features, measure predictive targets and provides actionable prediction models [11].

Deep learning uses artificial intelligence to process large information and extract meaningful patterns based on domain knowledge. It processes the data in hierarchical architectures like the human brain for classification, feature extraction or representational learning without the need for human intervention [11]. Regarding that, it still has some issues including unavailability of the dataset, privacy and legal issues, dedicated medical experts, data interoperability, data standards and others more [12].

Convolutional Neural Network (CNN) is one of the outbreaks in the evolution of deep learning. It is a method that is based on a sliding filter that scans over the image and creates a layer that consists of image features [13]. Then, an activation function is performed on each filter to produce an output between 0 and 1 which indicates the activation state. Simply, the activation function in a neural network is used to change the state or the activation level of a neuron into an output signal [11, 13]. After that, the results from each filter are passed to the second layer where it groups multiple filters to one neuron. Hence, the number of inputs in each neuron is fixed for all neurons. This process is repeated until the whole image is covered.

There are many activation functions developed and used in deep learning such as Rectified Linear Unit (ReLU), sigmoid and softmax. Moreover, Rectified Linear Unit (ReLU) is an activation function usually combines with other activation functions in order to get rid of negative numbers and exchange them with zeros [13]. Also, it helps retaining converged values instead of having a clog at a certain edge [13]. In fact, the ReLU function gained its reputation for that reason. That is, having converged values helps the machine to differentiate different values and classify data. The ReLU function can be represented with the following function [13]:

$$f(x) = \max(x, 0) \tag{1}$$

Where x is the number of inputs.

Sigmoid function is a non-linear function that is mostly used for the purpose of training data. Hence, it provides and output of either 0 or 1 [12]. Consequently, it is very useful in designing and understanding neural activity. It can be represented with the following function [12]:

$$f(s) = \frac{1}{(1 + e^{-x})} \tag{2}$$

Where x is the number of inputs.

Softmax is another popular activation function used for developing neural network models. Simply, it maps each output in a way that the total sum of a neuron is 1. Hence, the output is a probability distribution [13]. Consequently, the softmax function is mostly used in CNN. Softmax can be represented with the following function [13]:

$$\partial(z)_j = \frac{e^{zj}}{\sum_{k=1}^{K} e^{zk}} \text{for } j = 1, \ldots, k \tag{2}$$

Where z is a vector of inputs to outputs layer and j is the output units from 1 to k.

2.3 Image Processing

When talking about image processing, it is concerned with different techniques that generate a new array of numbers where it represents an enhanced image or classification of an image [13]. Whereas, image classification is a product of feature extraction techniques implemented using deep learning approaches. Although, some images can be difficult to analyze due to haziness or having a low resolution. Thus, preprocessing techniques can be applied to enhance image quality and remove any distortion or noises [14]. See Fig. 2.

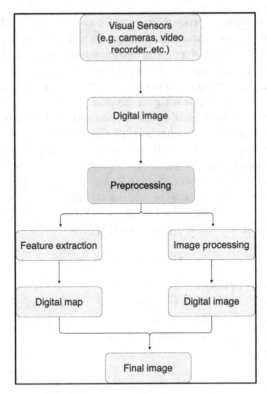

Fig. 2. Processes of image processing

The only way to detect diabetic retinopathy is through fundus images. That is, its complications are inside the retina tissue and cannot be visible by the naked eye. As mentioned before, these complications are exudates, microaneurysms and hemorrhages. Thus, many solutions have been developed using artificial intelligence and deep learning to process images and detect diabetic retinopathy for better classification and higher accuracy. And to diagnose diabetic retinopathy, its symptoms have to be detected and classified.

3   Related Work

In the past several years, the number of diabetic patients has increased in the world with an estimation of 463 million adults. Along with this chronic disease comes the possibility of being diagnosed with diabetic retinopathy. Since it can be early detected, there is a possibility of preventing or treating it. Therefore, many image processing techniques have been developed to detect and classify this disease in the early stages.

In [15], the authors used deep neural networks in the medical image to extract the information using the Siamese convolutional neural network (SCNN). Particularly, the method trains a pair of binary images that require less supervision. Also, they used a diabetic retinopathy fundus image dataset to evaluate their method. The researchers have provided a comparison between their state-of-the-art approach and a single supervised CNN approach which showed that their method required less supervision for training. Yet, they need to do more experiments on different metrics for evaluation like recall on top-N.

Where researchers in [11] have developed a deep learning approach using Convolutional Neural Network (CNN) for detecting diabetic retinopathy and fundus images as a dataset. Also, their approach has scored 97% sensitivity. As for [12], they used smartphone-based fundus photography and artificial intelligence to detect diabetic retinopathy. For the dataset, they used retinal photography of type 2 diabetes only. Furthermore, they used a software called EyeArtTM for detecting diabetic retinopathy. Consequently, the software scored a sensitivity of 95.8% and specificity of 80.2%.

As for in [16], a combination of fractal analysis and K-nearest neighbor (KNN) components have been used. This approach has scored an accuracy of 98.17%. Additionally, they used a Support Vector Machine (SVM) approach which separates blood vessels, exudates and microaneurysms for feature extraction and then, it detects the existence of diabetic retinopathy. This approach has scored 95% as maximum sensitivity.

4 Methodology

In the proposed approach, a deep learning technique was developed to detect diabetic retinopathy disease based on image processing using Python. On that account, our method is based on the Convolution Neural Networks (CNN) approach using fundus images. Thus, we used a MacOS operating system that uses a 1.8 GHz Intel Core i-5 processor, 8 GB memory.

CNN is known to be a supervised neural network. Hence, images were labeled based on the severity of the disease for classification. So first, the model takes fundus images as an input. Then, these images are pre-processed by being resized, padded, filtered and dilated. Hence, these operations are used to enhance images and improve feature extraction and classification. After that, images are segmented to locate boundaries and objects of each image. Thus, these segmentations are used for blood vessels, exudates, hemorrhage and microaneurysms detection. Then, the features of each label are extracted and images are classified based on disease severity. See Fig. 3.

4.1 Data Collection

In this study, a publicly available high-quality dataset from two databases were used. For the first dataset, the same dataset tested in [17] from GitHub was used. While the second dataset was taken from Kaggle [18]. Consequently, the dataset contained 600 fundus images for healthy patients and patients with diabetic retinopathy. Then, images were labeled based on the diabetic retinopathy stage whether it was not detected, low, mild or severe.

4.2 Preprocessing

For the preprocessing stage, re-sizing, interpolation, filtering and morphological operations were used to have a better visual of exudates, hemorrhage and microaneurysms.

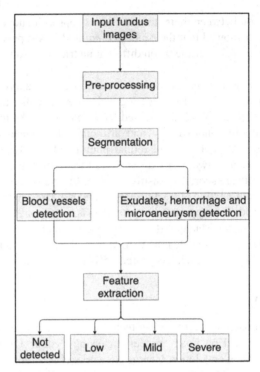

Fig. 3. Processes of the proposed model.

First, all images were re-sized to 90 × 90 pixels since images differed in size. Then, a bicubic interpolation was performed which takes 4 × 4 pixels to fill the neighboring pixels. After that, a median filter is performed to enhance the image. Finally, we used a morphological operation called dilation which adds pixels to the boundaries of an object in the image. Moreover, Fig. 4 shows a preprocessed image of a healthy eye where boundaries of the eye and retina veins are more visible but no sign of diabetic retinopathy was detected. As in Fig. 5, hemorrhage and exudates are much clearer and easier to detect.

4.3   Feature Extraction and Classification Using Deep Learning

After preprocessing, CNN was applied along with a window size of 3 × 3. Also, ReLU activation function was used for feature learning. While sigmoid function was used for feature extraction. In addition, the ReLU function was performed on each filter to produce an output between 0 and 1 at each neuron which finally provided the activation state and produced features of each label [19]. For the sigmoid function, it was used to provide an output of either 0 or 1 as well [20]. However, the final result of sigmoid function is the feature extraction for images. After that, we specified the input size to be 32 at each layer. Further, 90% of the dataset was used for training and 10% for validation.

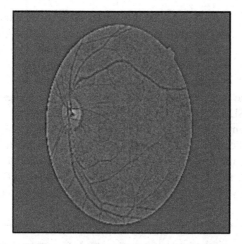

Fig. 4. Preprocessed fundus image of a healthy eye.

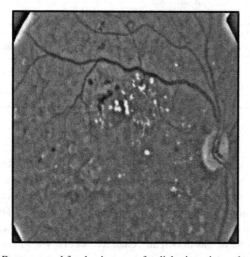

Fig. 5. Preprocessed fundus images of a diabetic retinopathy patient.

5 Results and Discussion

In preprocessing, resizing and applying gaussian filters on images were first applied. However, it produced a very low accuracy. Using different metrices, the processing of the images hit accuracy of 48% at best. Thus, the preprocessing technique was changed to median filter, morphology and interpolation. Thus, the resulted accuracy was much better.

During the testing phase, multiple parameters were experimented to increase the accuracy of the proposed method. Thus, a various types of activation functions were used along with manipulations of input size and validation dataset percentage. Hence, an experimentation of using softmax activation function in the feature extraction layer was done. However, the accuracy ranged from 40–50%. After experimenting with the sigmoid function, accuracy results have increased the by 50–80%. Further, using a large input size provided very poor outcomes. After multiple trials, an input size of 32 suited the proposed method. Also, an experimentation of varying the validation dataset from 10% to 30% was performed but it did not affect the accuracy rate.

With an input size of 32 and setting the epoch to 50, the highest accuracy achieved was 92.26% with MSE of 0.0628. See Fig. 6. Hence, it shows that the proposed method was successful in identifying diabetic retinopathy. Nonetheless, diabetic retinopathy is a serious disease that cannot be diagnosed at early stages. For that reason, more experimentation on enhancing this method could possibly done to obtain a higher accuracy. For example, Asymmetric CNN (ACNN) can be used to see its effect on the diagnosis of diabetic retinopathy since it is a promising method in image processing.

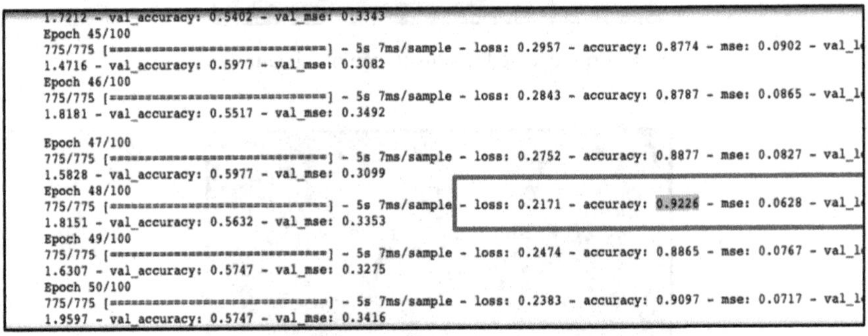

Fig. 6. Highest accuracy obtained.

Table 1 shows a comparison of the proposed technique and other techniques discussed in Sect. 3. Whereas, the proposed system scored higher accuracy than EyeArtTM system. However, the system proposed in [11] provided a better accuracy. Although, the method was not clearly explained in the preprocessing and classification. Thus, it is difficult to compare between the two approaches. KNN has also scored higher accuracy. According to the authors, using SVM has drastically changed accuracy for their technique. Hence, it can be used in the future to test it with the proposed system and test its potentials.

Table 1. A comparison between the proposed system and other diabetic retinopathy detection techniques.

Technique	Classification	Accuracy
Proposed system	CNN	92.26%
Razzak, M. I., Naz, S., Zaib, A. [11]	CNN	97%
Chung Y.A., Weng, W.H. [12]	EyeArtTM	80.02%
Schowengerdt, R. A. [16]	KNN	98.17%

6 Conclusion

Diabetic retinopathy is a serious disease that affects people with diabetes. Consequently, it is considered to be the most common cause of blindness among adults. Therefore, diabetic patients are required to do an annual check since it does not have any early symptoms. To assess the diagnosis of this disease, an image processing technique was proposed which uses CNN to detect diabetic retinopathy using fundus images. Additionally, a dataset from Kaggle and GitHub were used for the fundus images. To preprocess and enhance fundus image, morphological operations and normalization techniques were performed. Thus, the morphological operations used were: opening, closing, erosion and dilation. After that, the CNN technique was applied for image classification. As a result, the best accuracy obtained was of 92.26% with MSE of 0.0628. Hence, the results show promising results in detecting such serious disease with a prospect of improving.

References

1. Solomon, S.D., et al.: Erratum. diabetic retinopathy: a position statement by the American diabetes association. Diabetes Care **40**(6), 412–148 (2017)
2. Carrera, E.V., Gonzalez, A., Carrera, R.: Automated detection of diabetic retinopathy using SVM. In: IEEE XXIV International Conference on Electronics, Electrical Engineering and Computing (2017)
3. Khojasteh, P., Aliahmad, B., Kumar, D.K.: Fundus images analysis using deep features for detection of exudates, hemorrhages and microaneurysms. BMC Ophthalmol. **18**(1) (2018). https://doi.org/10.1186/s12886-018-0954-4
4. Rajalakshmi, R., Subashini, R., Anjana, R.M., Mohan, V.: Automated diabetic retinopathy detection in smartphone-based fundus photography using artificial intelligence. Eye **32**(6), 1138–1144 (2018)
5. Ray, S., Adhikary, P., Chatterjee, S., Midya, P., Palui, R., Ghosh, S.: A review on measurement of different parameters from retinal images to detect Glaucoma and Cataract. In: 2019 3rd International Conference on Electronics, Materials Engineering & Nano-Technology, IEMENTech (2019)
6. International Diabetes Federation Home. https://www.idf.org/our-network/regions-members.html. Accessed 8 Oct 2020
7. Saeedi, P., et al.: Global and regional diabetes prevalence estimates for 2019 and projections for 2030 and 2045: results from the International Diabetes Federation Diabetes Atlas, 9th edition. Diabetes Res. Clin. Pract. **157**, 107843 (2019)
8. Technology, A.: Cataract by Vessel Extraction from Fundus Images, pp. 638–641 (2017)
9. Kazi, A., Ajmera, M., Sukhija, P., Devadkar, K.: Processing retinal images to discover diseases. In: International Conference Current Trends Towards Converging Technology, ICCTCT 2018, pp. 1–5 (2018)
10. Goh, J.H.L., et al.: Artificial intelligence for cataract detection and management. Asia-Pacific J. Ophthalmol. **9**(2), 88–95 (2020)
11. Razzak, M.I., Naz, S., Zaib, A.: Deep learning for medical image processing: overview, challenges and the future. Lect. Notes Comput. Visual. BioApps **26**, 323–350 (2018)
12. Chung Y.A., Weng, W.H.: Learning Deep Representations of Medical Images using Siamese CNNs with Application to Content-Based Image Retrieval. arXiv, pp. 1–8 (2017)
13. Mitra, V., Franco, H.: Time-frequency convolutional networks for robust speech recognition. In: 2015 IEEE Workshop on Automatic Speech Recognition and Understanding (ASRU) (2015)

14. Liyakathunisa, Kumar C.N., Ananthashayana, V.K.: Super resolution reconstruction of low-resolution images using wavelet lifting schemes. Proc. ICCEE **9** (2009)

15. Wan, J.: Institutional Knowledge at Singapore Management University Deep learning for content-based image retrieval: a comprehensive study Chinese Academy of Sciences (2014)

16. Schowengerdt, R.A.: Techniques for Image Processing and Classifications in Remote Sensing. Academic press (2012)

17. Sejnowski, T.J.: The Deep Learning Revolution. MIT Press, London, England (2018)

18. Medium Activation functions: Sigmoid, ReLU, leaky ReLU and softmax basics for neural networks and deep learning. http://medium.com/@himanshuxd/activation-functions-sigmoid-relu-leaky-relu-and-softmax-basics-for-neural-networks-and-deep-8d9c70eed91e. Accessed 11 Dec 2020

19. Neural Network Concepts 7 types of activation functions in neural networks: how to choose? http://missinglink.ai/guides/neural-network-concepts/7-types-neural-network-activation-functions-right/. Accessed 11 Dec 2020

20. Sigmoid Function. Sciencedirect.com. https://www.sciencedirect.com/topics/computer-science/sigmoid-function. Accessed 24 Jun 2021

Automatic Classification of Diabetic Retinopathy Through Segmentation Using CNN

Saif Hameed Abbood[1,2]([envelope]) [ID], Haza Nuzly Abdull Hamed[1] [ID],
and Mohd Shafry Mohd Rahim[1] [ID]

[1] School of Computing, Faculty of Engineering, University Technology Malaysia (UTM),
81310 Johor, Malaysia
`saifhameed.it@gmail.com`, {`haza,shafry`}`@utm.my`
[2] Information Technology, Wasit Health Directorate, Iraqi Ministry of Health, 52001 Wasit, Iraq

Abstract. The process division of Diabetes Retinopathy (DR) has been considered as a significant step in diabetic retinopathy assessment and treatment. Different levels of microstructures like microaneurysm, rough exudates as well as neovascularization could take place on the retina area due to disruption to the retinal blood vessels triggered by elevated blood glucose levels. This is one of the primary causes of the prevalent visual impairment/blindness due to diabetes. Image segmentation, region merging, and Convolutional Neural Network (CNN) used in the paper for automated classification of high-resolution photographs of the retinal fundus in five stages of the DR. High heterogeneity is a significant problem for fundus image recognition for diabetic retinopathy, whereby new blood vessel proliferation including retinal detachment occurs. Therefore, careful examination of the retinal vessels is important to obtain accurate results which, through retinal segmentation could be achieved. We also highlight the difficulties in the development and learning of powerful, efficient, and reliable deep learning models for different DR diagnostic problems. The system was able to classify various DR stages with an average accuracy of around 94.2%, a sensitivity of 97%, and a specificity of 96%. There appears to be a genuine necessity for a steady interpretable classification system for DR and diabetic macular edema supported with solid confirmation. The suggested interpretable categorization systems allow diabetic retinopathy and macular edema to be properly classified. These technologies are expected to be beneficial in increasing diabetes screening and communication and discussion among those who care for these patients.

Keywords: Diabetic retinopathy · Computer vision · Image classification · Deep learning · Artificial intelligence

1 Introduction

Diabetic retinopathy (DR) is the leading cause of avoidable visual loss in people of working age in developed countries. The disease's global prevalence is estimated to rise at an exponential rate, reaching 529 million by 2030 [1]. As the number of persons diagnosed with diabetes rises, so does the number of people who get retinopathy.

S. Spinsante et al. (Eds.): HealthyIoT 2021, LNICST 432, pp. 99–112, 2022.
https://doi.org/10.1007/978-3-030-99197-5_9

This is concerning for worldwide national health care, as it affects people's ability to work, putting the economy in jeopardy. As a result, it is vital to provide a cost-effective and successful method of screening patients, which, when combined with collaborative treatment, has been credited with lowering the incidence of legal blindness in the working-age population [2].

The retina, which is spherical in shape, consists of a small membrane in the back of the eye. The purpose of the retina is to pass light into the neuronal signals as well as to communicate the sensory visual input with the brain 1. The retina is located next to the optic nerve, as well as a dark circular section present in the central region of the retina is known as the macula. The fovea is a key component of the macula that offers a clear sight [4].

Diabetic retinopathy (DR) is a diabetes complication that swells and drains fluids and blood from the veins of the retina [5]. If diabetic retinopathy, shifts to an advanced stage it can lead to vision loss. DR causes 2.6% of blindness worldwide [6]. In diabetic patients with a long-term illness, the risk of diabetes retinopathy rises. Normal retinal screening is critical for the diagnosis and early treatment of DR in patients with diabetes to prevent blindness [7]. The presence of various forms of lesions in a retina picture is determined by diabetic retinopathy. These lesions are soft and hard Exudates (EXs), Hemorrhages (HMs), and Microaneurysms (MAs) [8, 9].

The presence of excessive blood glucose in the blood develops diabetic retinopathy and affects minute blood vessels within the retina. These tiny blood vessels will leak fluids and blood into the retina, which will form characteristics such as hemorrhages, micro-aneurysms, spots of cotton wool, rough exudates, vein loops, macula swelling, and thickening [10]. Moreover, as blood flow is being supplied, the retina begins to develop several new abnormally fragile blood vessels called Intraretinal Microvascular Abnormalities IrMAs [11]. Non-Proliferative DR (NPDR) and Proliferative DR can be commonly called (PDR) [5]. The phases of DR may be graded depending on the appearance of characteristic features on the retinal fundus.

The elevated pressure in the eye could cause late-stage damage to the optic nerve. Therefore, DR can be indicated momentarily as a lack of vision (which in this situation is irreversible) due to symptoms of diabetes of retinal blood vessels. Exudates [12] are a crucial symptom of diabetic retinopathy that can be bagged in a picture of the retinal fundus and is the evidence for the production or development of the DR in the patient. Retinal testing for weakened eyes at the early stages is a potential solution for diagnosis (Fig. 1) [13].

Early detection of diabetic retinopathy can minimize vision acuity, visual impairment, and related morbidity [15]. Early diagnosis may lower the risks of DR. The most prevalent vision-threatening lesions in Type 1 diabetes are the Proliferative Diabetic Retinopathy (PDR) as well as the most prominent Type 2 disorder is Diabetic Macular Edema (DME) which significantly result in mild visual losses. The retinal fundus tests allow the retinal vasculature as well as underlying anatomy to be specifically visualized. Retinal vasculature disruption is largely due to the pathogenicity and clinical characteristics of DR. In the early stages the DR identification may also help in the diagnosis of developing lesions through retinal fundus images [16].

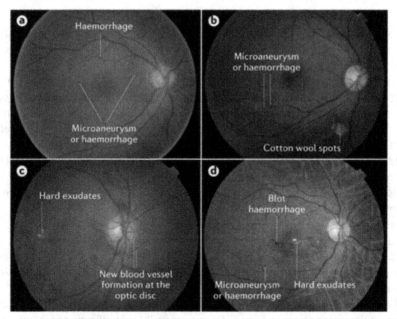

Fig. 1. Fundus images showing various DR developments (a–d) (Source: Nature Reviews/Disease Primers) [14]

Various approaches could be adopted to diagnose diabetic retinopathy. Usually, the retinal fundus is examined by an ophthalmologist with a pupil dilatation, whether with an indirect ophthalmoscope or slit-light biomicroscope [17]. Put another way, a dilated pupil assists in taking photographs of the fundus, and afterward, these images can be investigated by an ophthalmologist. The state-of-the-art in diabetic retinopathic diagnosis is the Early Treatment of Diabetic Retinopathy Study (ETDRS), performed by professional photograms and skilled ophthalmologists, using 30°, 7 standard field stereoscopy 35 mm (7F-ETDRS) color slides or with the help of fundus fluorescein angiography (FFA) [18].

Telemedicine is increasingly used to diagnose diabetic retinopathy and, in particular, to scan for the DR on basis of digital images from retinal fundus compressed (or otherwise), processed and sent to a distant ophthalmologist for further evaluations [19]. Through the extraction and classification of characteristics, segmentation may be utilized in medical research to separate various tissues from one another [20, 21].

The purpose and contribution of this work are achieving a high accuracy classification of five diabetic retinopathy stages as an aim to simulate the clinical diagnosis of the expert ophthalmologists.

2   Literature Review

The current medical imaging literature review provides promising outcomes in various modalities of medical scanning and imagery [22]. Salehinejad et al. [23] suggested the development of X-rays for the identification of chest Disorders by a Convolutionary Generative Adversarial Networks (DC-GAN). They demonstrated that artificial data is better than the actual unbalanced and balanced data sets as well as it improves the detection performances and accuracies.

Rad A. E. [24] devised a methodology for analyzing dental x-ray pictures and diagnosing caries problems in teeth Enhancement was used to increase the quality of the X-ray pictures, and the Thresholding approach was used to make the pictures simpler. The individual tooth was extracted using the integral projection approach, and a feature map of the tooth surface was created for the analysis and detection procedure.

Mazhar J. Awan [25] presented a method for Knee Anterior Cruciate Ligament from Magnetic Resonance Imaging by combining class balance and data augmentation, a 14-layer ResNet-14 convolutional neural network (CNN) architecture with six alternative orientations.

The relevance and viability of diabetic retinopathy diagnosis telemedicine were assessed by Vaziri et al. [26], as a predictor, with a standard statistical consensus value (κ statistics). The goal of this analysis was to evaluate the telemedicine and classification precision within the full scope of DR and Diabetic Macular Edema (DME) in comparison to today's gold standards.

The previous research in the identification of different phases of diabetic retinopathy focused on the systematic extraction of features as well as classification of features using different techniques of computer vision & machine learning-based classification models. Rahim et al. [27] published a 2016 approach for the use of blurred picture treatment for diabetic retinopathy. Method focused on the different lesions of the retinal tract including the hemorrhages, exudates, micro-aneurysms, blood vessels, etc.

A method to automatically diagnose non-proliferative DR was suggested by Al-Jarrah and Shatnawi in [28]. The approach was based upon the identification of MAs and HAs by extracting essential features including the optic disks, fovea as well as blood vessels to accurately segment the lesions of the dark spot.

Yi-Peng Liu [29] WP-CNN was presented, which was motivated by ensemble learning. Backpropagation is used to optimize various path weight coefficients, and the output features are averaged for redundancy reduction and fast convergence in WP-CNN.

An ensemble for classifying the retinal image suggested by Balazs Harangi [30] that combines a convolutional neural network (CNN) with traditional hand-crafted features into a single design. To offer a final forecast, this method combines CNN training with fine-tuning of the weights of handcrafted characteristics. This solution is focused on automatically classifying fundus images based on the severity of DR and DME.

Gautami ghan [31] suggested a model to diagnose DR from digital anatomical structure images, the methodology uses the R-CNN (Regional Convolutional Neural Network) approach. The complete image is segmented in the suggested method, and the regions of interest are extracted for further processing. The suggested method employs four layers of convolutional neural networks to train 130 anatomical features and is then tested on 100 photos. All of the photographs are divided into two categories: those with DR and those without.

Iyyanar P [32] presented a CNN approach for automatic classification of diabetic retinopathy through spatial analysis, The proposed approach is to create a more efficient and effective way to identify images using minimal pre-processing procedures.

These methods perform slightly worse than earlier methods, owing to the failure of the neural network to learn critical aspects such as the proliferation of new blood vessels and retinal detachment that occur during the lateral phases of diabetic retinopathy with a high severity level.

According to our study of the previous work, some limitations are noticed in that approached such as the methods which were used in some works are not achieved high accuracies [29–31], in addition, some works such as [26–28] are not detected all lesions of diabetic retinopathy such us neovascular of the retina that's mean not all stages of diabetic retinopathy are detected, this shows the necessity of more researches in the field to achieve high accuracies to simulate the clinical diagnosis of disease.

We utilized U-Net segmentation in this work with region merging and a Convolutional Neural Network to detect the various phases of Diabetic Retinopathy. The technique of automatically detecting the borders of blood vessels within the retina is known as retinal segmentation. This helps the classifier to pick up on essential characteristics like retinal growth and separation. Through region merging, losing data is very expected in the segmentation stage owing to the incorporation of retinal segmentation. This technique exceeds previous approaches by a factor of 94.2% ACC, furthermore, for each class, we create important score pixel-maps to assist experienced ophthalmologists to deduce as well as comprehend the outcomes.

3 Methodology

Fundus photography is an imaging technique widely applied to record the scope of disease in medical diagnostic settings and clinical trials. The picture of the fundus consists of 3 channels: red, green, and blue (RGB). Moreover, the retinal fundus images contain three types: color fundus, red-free, and stereo fundus. The DR characteristics, including intra-retinal hemorrhagic structures, microaneurysms, wedged cotton-wool spots, virulence beading, extensive growth of blood vessels, and Intra-retinal Microvascular Abnormalities (IrMA) have been described by seven standard color fundus images. Digital retinal fundus images are a fast-imaging technique that can be accessed in a highly availability, non-invasively, and well-tolerated fashion.

High variability, particularly for proliferative DR within which, the retinal spread of new blood vessels including retinal separation occurs, is an important problem in the diagnosis of fundus photos. The method of automated identification of blood vessel boundaries is known as retinal segmentation. Therefore, we must locate the position and emergence of the new blood vessel to calculate the retinal feature extraction through image segmentation (Fig. 2 and Fig. 3). The correct examination of the retinal blood vessels is important to obtain the exact results, that could be accomplished by retinal segmentation. As mentioned, retinal segmentation is an automated blood vessel boundary detection mechanism.

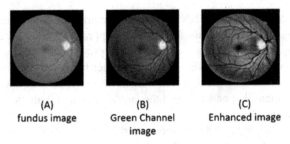

(A)
fundus image

(B)
Green Channel
image

(C)
Enhanced image

Fig. 2. Fundus image pre-processing and enhancement [33] (Color figure online)

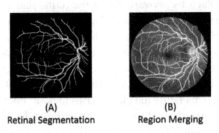

(A)
Retinal Segmentation

(B)
Region Merging

Fig. 3. Fundus image segmentation [33]

3.1 Proposed Method

The approach presented in this paper intends at the detection of the different phases of DR via retinal segmentations with U-Net along with the merging of the region & using convolutional neural networks. Retina segmentation is the mechanism by which the blood vessel boundary inside the retina is automatically detected. This helps classificatory predictors to learn essential features like the proliferation of retina as well as retinal detachments. The data lost in the event of segmentation of the retinal image is restored using region merging (Fig. 4).

The U-net Framework is an encoding-decoding paradigm that has some skip interfaces between the decoder and the encoder modules. This architectural design's key benefit is that it can take a broader context into consideration when planning for a pixel-based predictor.

Preprocessing, Retinal Segmentation, and Classifier are the three stages of the approach proposed in this paper. In Fig. 4, the proposed method's flowchart is depicted. The database comprises high-resolution retina fundus photographs with a large black boundary. As shown in Fig. 2(A), we started by removing the majority of the black borders and then resizing the photos to 480 × 480 pixels. Data augmentation is the most effective way to avoid overfitting. Image transformations such as color augmentation, translation, rotation, flipping, stretching, are used in the augmentation step. The training set is increased by an element of two thanks to the data augmentation. The network suffers from significant overfitting without data augmentation. The fundus picture has three channels: red, green, and blue. To calculate the segmentation of the retina, we must monitor the location of the blood vessels. When compared to a brighter background, the darker blood vessels contrast refines substantially. As seen in Fig. 2(B), the stronger

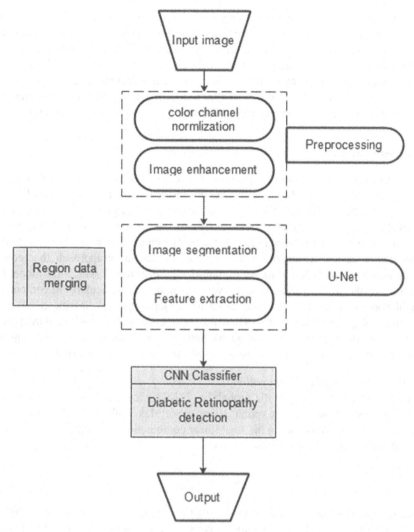

Fig. 4. Process for automatic DR detection

green portion enhanced the contrast of the retinal image, resulting in the best outcome. As an outcome, we chose the green channel of an image and sent it to be preprocessed further, after enhancement, these images are fed into U-net, which performs retinal segmentation. Figure 2(C) depicts the outcome of picture enhancement.

The technique of automatically detecting the borders of blood vessels within the retina is known as retinal segmentation. This enables the classifier to pick up on critical characteristics like retinal detachment and retinal proliferation. These characteristics play a crucial role in the characterization of diabetic retinopathy and considerably increase accuracy. The retinal segmentation was done with the use of a neural network. The U-Net is a Convolutional Neuron network with an imminent and advancing path in its architecture. The approaching path captures context and is symmetric, whereas the advancing path allows for exact localize. This is the best way way to do retinal segmentation. Figure 3(A) shows the result of retinal segmentation. As illustrated in Fig. 3(B), to recover data lost during retinal segmentation, the U-output Net is subsequently subjected to region merging with its input image. The classifier is a convolutional neural network that learns features of pictures produced after retinal segmentation with region merging and uses them to classify diabetic retinopathy into five stages based on severity.

3.2 Deep Learning

Deep Learning (DL) techniques [34] in several automated classification-based problems have already been employed commonly over the past few years. For image classification, the normal method involves extraction of the essential characteristics from a collection of convolutionary layers, which is followed by a final grading by a group of fully convolution layers with those characteristic attributes. The parametric values are modified in the training process while utilizing a gradient-based optimization approach, that reduces a predetermined loss function to a minimum [35]. After the classification model has been trained (the parameters of model layers are adjusted), particularly in comparison with the correct "true" values contained in a labeled dataset where classification quality determines the performance quality. These data are regarded as the gold standard, preferably based on the expertise of a human specialist's panel. Further, the image mapping enables multi-dimensional items to be grouped into a smaller number of classes.

Classification of Diabetic Retinopathy

The proposed model estimates the probability P(K|I) since C belongs to the potential class of production and I to the retina. Using a SoftMax method [36] as a final layer upon the given values following the final linear combination of selected features. This can be determined as the probability function:

$$P(K/I)_i = e^{Z_i} / \sum_{j=1}^{C} e^{Z_j} \tag{1}$$

Before using SoftMax, let us consider the final value of any output neuron, which is for instance calculated as ZK for the Class K ranking. To measure the likelihood of all groups, we need a normalization function from SoftMax, however, in this event, we just want to test SoftMax within the context of argmax (SoftMax), since argmax (Zi) = argmax (SoftMax (Zi)). Therefore, we ignore SoftMax from within the assessment of class definition.

Dataset

The data collection consisted of the retinal fundus downloaded from Kaggle (containing about 67k images) for the training/testing of diabetic retinopathy. Other patient information (demographic profile) was not used in the present data sets. In each of the images, various DR stages, as well as severeness of the symptoms, were measured. In this paper, the International Clinical Diabetic Retinopathy (ICDR) scores were used for the classification and grading of DR using retinal fundus images [37], which indicates no/normal

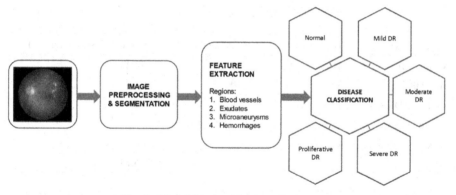

Fig. 5. Model for classification of DR stages

DR (0), moderate DR (1), mild DR (2), severe DR (3) and proliferative DR (4). Figure 5 represents the model for the classification of DR stages.

Consequently, around 207 retinal fundus images from the EyePACS database collection of Kaggle were collected for this analysis. For the training and validation algorithm, 70% maculation-centered images from the dataset were used (referred to as development set, divided into training (~68%) and tuning set (~2%)). We also used 30% of the dataset as test data to measure the algorithm's output to determine the performance of the algorithm.

Convolutional Neural Network (CNN)
Convolutional Neural Network CNNs are more effective algorithmically and in computational integrity than full connected networks. Therefore, CNNs are perfect to take advantage of the general high-local image correlations and the pixel mapping.

4 Results

The output of the model was found to predict various stages of diabetic retinopathy based on hemorrhages, exudates/hard exudates, proliferative blood vessels, microaneurysm, cotton wool spots, etc. Table 1 shows the outputs of the present classification model for diabetic retinopathy. The findings reveal that the classification model makes the precise estimation of the unspecified class efficiently with about 85% accuracy. It was able to accurately forecast severe DR (3), moderate DR (2), mild DR (1), as well as Proliferative DR (4) up, to 86%, 81%, 92.04%, and 88.72%, respectively. The classification model reported an 82% sensitivity, an 86% accuracy as well as up to 95% high prediction efficiency. Figure 6 and Fig. 7 show classification results of DR predictions. Figure 8 represents the plotting curve for training and testing via model.

Table 1. DR classification results

Stage (class)	Training dataset	Testing dataset	Correct classification (%)
Normal (0)	41	8	84.43
Mild DR (1)	50	10	81
Moderate DR (2)	49	8	92.04
Severe DR (3)	53	10	86
PDR (4)	41	8	88.72
Mean			86.74

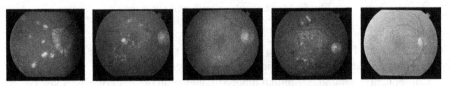

Fig. 6. Classification of DR (Test 1)

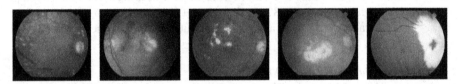

Fig. 7. Classification of DR stages (Test 2)

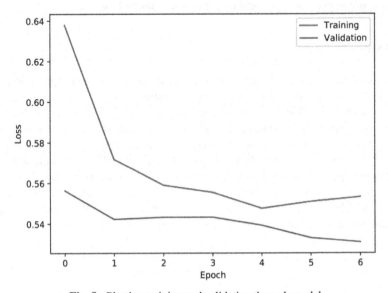

Fig. 8. Plotting training and validation through model

Table 2 below, represents a salient comparison among previous works based on method, accuracy, sensitivity, and specificity.

Table 2. Comparison of previous works

Reference	Classes	Method	Accuracy (%)	Sensitivity (%)	Specificity (%)
[12]	3	Blood vessels, exudates, and texture	93.6	90.3	100
[15]	2	Decision support system	–	100	63
[26]	5	Higher order spectra	82	82.5	88.9
[27]	4	Area of blood vessels, exudates	84	91.7	100
[34]	2	Hemorrhages, blood vessels, microaneurysms, exudates	–	74.8	82.7
[30]	5	Hemorrhages, exudates, blood vessels, microaneurysms,	90.07		
[31]	5	Hemorrhages, exudates, blood vessels, microaneurysms,	93		
[32]	5	Hemorrhages, exudates, blood vessels, microaneurysms,	90		
Proposed work	5	Hemorrhages, exudates, blood vessels, microaneurysms,	94.2	97	96

According to the comparison Table 2 between the previous models with current U-Net, the methods [12, 15, 26, 27] which achieved good results have not detected all features of five stages of diabetic retinopathy such as [12] extracted 3 classes only with 93.6% ACC, as well as [27], while the methods [30–32, 34] detected all features, however, it couldn't achieve high results in comparison with the current work which is achieved high results and all features detection, are achieved 90.07%, 93%, 90%, respectively. The proposed regional model has a higher level of accuracy. This is because

DR lesions were extracted from regional features. U-Net assists in the extraction of additional useful features for classification.

Among all the networks on the test set, the proposed U-Net technique has the best accuracy rate of 94.2%. We also look at the sensitivity and specificity indexes for the prediction result to see how well the model performs on the referable diabetic retinopathy identification task. The identification system threshold in clinical diagnosis can be modified according to the diagnosis requirement for expected sensitivity and specificity. As a result, because it indicates the prediction confidence degree, which shows the model generalization power, it is an important quantitative statistic in practical application. The best result is achieved by our U-Net model, showing that the suggested network has greater classification performance and confidence.

5 Conclusion and Future Work

The paper proposed an optimal model for Diabetic Retinopathy detection, we used U-Net approach to design this model. It was also observed that preprocessing of DR images is very essential to get proper features. In the case of noisy images, the chances of getting poor data will lead to lower accuracies. Additionally, we applied the model with image pre-processing for an interpretable DR classifier, achieving more than 94% of accuracy for the detection of various classes of diabetic retinopathy. The system was able to classify various DR stages with an average accuracy of around 94.2%, a sensitivity of 97%, and a specificity of 96%. The proposed framework not only allows retinal fundus images to be classified in 5 ICDR standardized DR grades, but it can also produce significant score pixel-maps for each class to allow professional ophthalmologists to deduce as well as perceive the results. Automated tools have the potential to improve the quality of DR screening, increase access to health care, and lower the cost of screening. Early detection and therapy may assist to avoid the beginning of the disease or slow the progression of the condition. In the future, the automated network design based on feature amalgamation will receive increasing attention, also we are trying to use a generative adversarial network to solve the lack and imbalance of data and try to train the networks using a limited amount of data.

References

1. Qureshi, I., Ma, J., Abbas, Q.: Recent development on detection methods for the diagnosis of diabetic retinopathy. Symmetry **11**, 749, (2019)
2. Liew, G., Michaelides, M., Bunce, C.: A comparison of the causes of blindness certifications in England and Wales in working-age adults (16–64 years), 1999–2000 with 2009–2010. BMJ Open **4**, e004015 (2014)
3. Fenner, B.J., Wong, R.L., Lam, W.C., Tan, G.S., Cheung, G.C.: Advances in retinal imaging and applications in diabetic retinopathy screening: a review. Ophthalmol. Therapy **7**(2), 333–346 (2018)
4. Li, X., Li, X.: The antidepressant effect of light therapy from retinal projections. Neurosci. Bull. **34**(2), 359–368 (2018)
5. Shi, L., Wu, H., Dong, J., Jiang, K., Lu, X., Shi, J.: Telemedicine for detecting diabetic retinopathy: a systematic review and meta-analysis. Br. J. Ophthalmol. **99**(6), 823–831 (2015)

6. Bourne, R.R., et al.: Causes of vision loss worldwide, 1990–2010: a systematic analysis. Lancet Glob. Health **1**(6), 339–349 (2013)
7. Chakrabarti, R., Harper, C.A., Keeffe, J.E.: Diabetic retinopathy management guidelines. Exp. Rev. Ophthal. **7**(5), 417–439 (2012)
8. Salz, D.A., Witkin, A.J.: Imaging in diabetic retinopathy. Middle East Afr. J. Ophthalmol. **22**(2), 145 (2015)
9. Bawankar, P., et al.: Sensitivity and specificity of automated analysis of single-field non-mydriatic fundus photographs by Bosch DR algorithm—comparison with mydriatic fundus photography (ETDRS) for screening in undiagnosed diabetic retinopathy. PLoS ONE **12**(12), e0189854 (2017)
10. Vo, H.H., Verma, A.: Discriminant color texture descriptors for diabetic retinopathy recognition. In: 2016 IEEE 12th International Conference on Intelligent Computer Communication and Processing (ICCP) 8 September 2016, pp. 309–315. IEEE (2016)
11. Gupta, G., Kulasekaran, S., Ram, K., Joshi, N., Sivaprakasam, M., Gandhi, R.: Local characterization of neovascularization and identification of proliferative diabetic retinopathy in retinal fundus images. Comput. Med. Imaging Graph. **55**, 124–132 (2017)
12. Patil, P., Shettar, P., Narayankar, P., Patil, M.: An efficient method of detecting exudates in diabetic retinopathy: using texture edge features. In: 2016 International Conference on Advances in Computing, Communications, and Informatics (ICACCI), pp. 1188–1191 (2016)
13. Prasad, D.K., Vibha, L, Venugopal, K.R.: Early detection of diabetic retinopathy from digital retinal fundus images. In 2015 IEEE Recent Advances in Intelligent Computational Systems (RAICS), 240–245 (2015)
14. Wong Ty, C.C., Larsen, M.: Sharma, S., Simo, R.: Diabetic retinopathy. Nat. Rev. Dis. Primers **2**, 16012 (2016)
15. Xu, K., Feng, D., Mi, H.: Deep convolutional neural network-based early automated detection of diabetic retinopathy using fundus image. Molecules **22**(12), 2054 (2017)
16. Winder, R.J., Morrow, P.J., McRitchie, I.N., Bailie, J.R., Hart, P.M.: Algorithms for digital image processing in diabetic retinopathy. Comput. Med. Imaging Graph. **33**(8), 608–622 (2009)
17. Wat, N., Wong, R.L., Wong, I.Y.: Associations between diabetic retinopathy and systemic risk factors. Hong Kong Med J. **22**(6), 589–599 (2016)
18. Chui, T.Y., et al.: Longitudinal imaging of microvascular remodeling in proliferative diabetic retinopathy using adaptive optics scanning light ophthalmoscopy. Ophthalmic Physiol. Opt. **36**(3), 290–302 (2016)
19. Cheloni, R., Gandolfi, S.A., Signorelli, C., Odone, A.: Global prevalence of diabetic retinopathy: protocol for a systematic review and meta-analysis. BMJ Open **9**(3), e022188 (2019)
20. Norouzi, A., et al.: Medical image segmentation methods, algorithms, and applications. IETE Tech. Rev. **31**(3), 199–213 (2014)
21. Sami, A.S., Rahim, M.S.M., Ahmed, F.Y.H., Sulong, G.B.: A review study of methods utilized for identifying and segmenting the brain tumor from MR imageries (2019)
22. Norouzi, A., et al.: Medical image segmentation methods, algorithms, and applications. IETE Tech. Rev. **31**(3), 199–213 (2014)
23. Salehinejad, H., Colak, E., Dowdell, T., Barfett, J., Valaee, S.: Synthesizing chest x-ray pathology for training deep convolutional neural networks. IEEE Trans. Med. Imaging **38**(5), 1197–1206 (2018)
24. Rad, A.E., Amin, I.B.M., Rahim, M.S.M., Kolivand, H.: Computer-aided dental caries detection system from X-ray images. In: Phon-Amnuaisuk, S., Au, T.W. (eds.) Computational Intelligence in Information Systems. AISC, vol. 331, pp. 233–243. Springer, Cham (2015). https://doi.org/10.1007/978-3-319-13153-5_23

25. Awan, M.J., Rahim, M.S.M., Salim, N., Mohammed, M.A., Garcia-Zapirain, B., Abdulka-reem, K.H.: Efficient detection of knee anterior cruciate ligament from magnetic resonance imaging using deep learning approach. Diagnostics (Basel) 11(1), 105 (2021)
26. Vaziri, K., Moshfeghi, D.M., Moshfeghi, A.A.: Feasibility of telemedicine in detecting diabetic retinopathy and age-related macular degeneration. In Seminars in ophthalmology. Inf. Healthcare 30(2), 81–95 (2015)
27. Rahim, S.S., Palade, V., Shuttleworth, J., Jayne, C.: Automatic screening and classification of diabetic retinopathy and maculopathy using fuzzy image processing. Brain Inform. 3(4), 249–267 (2016). https://doi.org/10.1007/s40708-016-0045-3
28. Al-Jarrah, M.A., Shatnawi, H.: Non-proliferative diabetic retinopathy symptoms detection and classification using neural network. J. Med. Eng. Technol. 41(6), 498–505 (2017)
29. Liu, Y.P, Li, Z., Xu, C., Li, J., Liang, R.: Referable diabetic retinopathy identification from eye fundus images with weighted path for convolutional neural network. Artif. Intell. Med. 99, 101694 (2019)
30. Harangi, B., Toth, J., Baran, A., Hajdu, A.: Automatic screening of fundus images using a combination of convolutional neural network and hand-crafted features. In: 2019 41st Annual International Conference of the IEEE Engineering in Medicine and Biology Society (EMBC), pp. 2699–2702 (2019)
31. Ghan, G., Chavan, S., Chaudhari, A.: Diabetic retinopathy classification using deep learning. In: Fourth International Conference on Inventive Systems and Control (ICISC), 2020, pp. 761–765 (2020)
32. Iyyanar, P., Parthasarathy, J.: Diabetic retinopathy classification using deep learning framework. J. Crit. Rev. 7(14), 2683–2689 (2020)
33. Adapa, D., Joseph Raj, A.N., Alisetti, S.N., Zhuang, Z., Naik, G.: A supervised blood vessel segmentation technique for digital Fundus images using Zernike Moment based features. PLoS ONE 15(3), e0229831 (2020)
34. Cao, P., Ren, F., Wan, C., Yang, J., Zaiane, O.: Efficient multi-kernel multi-instance learning using weakly supervised and imbalanced data for diabetic retinopathy diagnosis. Comput. Med. Imaging Graph. 1(69), 112–124 (2018)
35. Scanlon, P.H.: The English national screening program for diabetic retinopathy 2003–2016. Acta Diabetol. 54(6), 515–525 (2017)
36. Nwankpa, C., et al., Activation Functions: Comparison of trends in Practice and Research for Deep Learning. In: 2nd International Conference on Computational Sciences and Technology (INCCST) (2020)
37. Sahlsten, J., et al.: Deep learning fundus image analysis for diabetic retinopathy and macular edema grading. Sci. Rep. 9(1), 1–1 (2019)

Pulp Stone Detection Using Deep Learning Techniques

Amal Selmi, Liyakathunisa Syed, and Bashaer Abdulkareem$^{(\boxtimes)}$

Taibah University, Medina, Saudi Arabia
amal.alrehily@gmail.com, lansari@taibahu.edu.sa,
b.alhejaily@gmail.com

Abstract. Today, the aid of modern technology in the medical field can be seen in every respect. In the field of radiology, many deep learning and image processing techniques have been applied for timely and better analysis, as well as conclusive results. However, dental radiographs are detailed, and some of these details are fine and vague, making them difficult to interpret. With the help of deep learning techniques, the automated uncovering of these fine details has great potential. In this paper, we aim to detect pulp stones in dental radiographs using Convolutional Neural Network (CNN)-based feature extraction followed by multiple classifiers. We conclude that the Residual Network 50 (ResNet-50) achieves an accuracy of 76.4% with the Medium Gaussian Support Vector Machine (SVM), while Inception v3 reaches an accuracy of 73.1% with the same classifier. Further, the ResNet-50's false positive rate is less than the Inception v3's by 7%, giving it the potential for further experiments.

Keywords: Deep learning · Dental radiographs · Pulp stones · Convolutional Neural Networks · Medium Gaussian Support Vector Machine

1 Introduction

Image processing is one of the most important and utilised concepts of computer science and modern technology. Moreover, it is used in multiple applications such as industrial inspection, the military, remote sensing, and medical imaging [1]. Moreover, researchers began to focus on automated analysis for medical images as soon as images became digitised. Initially, the analysis of medical images was accomplished using sequential applications of mathematical modelling and low-level pixel processing to build compound systems that were rule-based and had the ability to solve specific tasks. Furthermore, Artificial Intelligence (AI) analogy using expert systems with a large number of if–then–else conditional statements were popular from the 1970s to the 1990s [2]. However, we witnessed a shift from human-designed systems to computer-trained systems that use example data to train and extract feature vectors. Training systems with data given in pairs of images and that correlate outcomes for the images are known as supervised learning [3]. Thus, supervised techniques gained increasing popularity in the analysis of medical images by the end of the 1990s [2].

© ICST Institute for Computer Sciences, Social Informatics and Telecommunications Engineering 2022
Published by Springer Nature Switzerland AG 2022. All Rights Reserved
S. Spinsante et al. (Eds.): HealthyIoT 2021, LNICST 432, pp. 113–124, 2022.
https://doi.org/10.1007/978-3-030-99197-5_10

In the medical field, AI techniques, and computer vision in particular, are applied widely. Additionally, deep learning using Convolutional Neural Networks (CNNs) is known as a type of the many models of machine learning and has proven to have astounding potential to assist doctors in the detection of pathologies. Moreover, it has the potential to detect bodily-related structures from medical images with high accuracy that can surpass that of medical professionals. CNNs also have the ability to detect structures (e.g., decide if a tooth is on an image), segment them (e.g., identify the precise shape of a tooth on an image) and classify them (e.g., label every tooth in a dentition) [3].

Undoubtedly, medical imaging plays a critical role in fields such as dentistry. Today, dentists diagnose patients by analysing the patient's panoramic radiographs. After that, they observe and register tooth conditions, such as those of implants, dental bridges etc. Additionally, the Federation Dentaire International notation system is used to register tooth symptoms, a process that uses Arabic numerals to clarify the positioning of the tooth. The dentition is then accurately divided into four quadrants, with eight teeth in each quadrant, and each tooth is identified by its two-digit number. The first of the two digits indicates the quadrant in which the tooth is located, while the second digit indicates the tooth's number in this quadrant. Overall, the assessment of the tooth conditions is through observation, and the recording is done manually in a text file. As a result, the full process costs considerable effort and time, with delays in diagnostic results [1] and obstructions to the clinic's workflow. Furthermore, some studies clarify that dentistry students' traditional way of interpreting radiographic images is inaccurate. Thus, we cannot depend on observation only to identify complex and vague cases [4]. Therefore, for a clinical decision support system that is based on imaging, medical image classification is a crucial step. However, the existing techniques for X-ray image classification present the image using only its generic features, such as its shape and colour. Hence, the ability to measure the image's characteristics is limited [5].

A large volume of images is acquired every year in the dental field. For example, in European countries, dental radiography such as panoramic and cephalometric radiography is likely the most taken type of radiograph in the medical field. For instance, it was roughly calculated that between 250 and 300 dental images for every 1000 individuals were taken in 2010. Additionally, CNNs in medicine have been successfully used for object detection in image segmentation and recognition, and recently, CNNs have been used in the field of dentistry to reveal periodontal bone loss [6]. Thus, the application of CNNs has much potential in the dentistry field, even though which CNN applications are most focused upon or which techniques (imagery types, outcome metrics etc.) are most popular has not been systematically assessed. Additionally, it is not clear how CNNs perform in comparison to human experts. Thus, further research and implementation could help to evaluate how advantageous the application of CNNs is for dental clinical practice [3].

Even though multiple CNN applications have been used in the dental field, such as cavity classification [8], oral cancer detection [9], teeth segmentation [10] etc., the detection of fine and vague objects such as pulp stones using radiography is yet to be explored. Therefore, in this paper, we aim to detect pulp stones in X-ray images using CNN-based feature extraction and the application of different classifiers.

The paper is organised as follows: background, methodology, experimentation, results and discussion and conclusion.

2 Background

2.1 Convolutional Neural Networks

CNN is a deep learning technique that implicitly extracts image data from deeper networks through feature extraction. Specifically, the CNN model consists of several layers of convolution and pooling that are stacked on top of each other. Additionally, several weights are shared by the convolutional layer, while the pooling layer sub-samples the convolutional layer output and reduces the data rate [15]. Additionally, CNN is commonly used in the area of image processing. Moreover, it has been inspired by biological processes such as the human brain's ability to distinguish between various objects through visuals only and the use of previous observations. This phenomenon can be used in the processing of medical images to classify various images and identify diseases [15].

2.2 Deep Learning in Dentistry

In 2017, research started to use CNN to detect teeth. In a study, the automated identification of teeth and their numbering was performed using CNN, and a heuristic approach was used to detect the teeth [16]. Structure identification and segmentation are the main tasks that CNNs have been tested for so far. Surprisingly, even with the given difficulties in dental image diagnostics, a few studies inspected the detection of pathologies resulting in limited accuracy and reliability. Seemingly, the focus of researchers has been on basic tasks such as identification (e.g., mostly tooth identification) because it is considered the foundation of more complex detection systems. Then, as a subsequent step, pathologies are detected and allocated to the teeth [3].

Schwendicke et al. (2019) the authors studied a collection of existing literature and concluded that almost half of the studies have used CNN architectures that are individually constructed. Furthermore, CNNs performed remarkably well when applied to medical imagery. Their application could allow for more thorough, precise and reliable disease detection and image evaluation. Notably, the use of CNNs has been continuously increasing in the field of dental research. However, even though the first published application for CNN in dentistry was in 2015, there is no significant leap in sight. On the other hand, medicine had 42 CNN entries available on PubMed in 2015 and over 800 in the first half of 2019. Therefore, it is likely that dentistry is following medicine in general in terms of the application of CNNs. Thus, this may allow for the clarification of methodological standards and early strictness, but different disciplines possess large amounts of evidence, which may lead to bias [3].

Many deep learning algorithms are composed of several layers that convert input data, such as images, into outputs, such as existing diseases. The use of CNNs is broadening presently in the analysis of medical images [2]. Lee et al. (2018) the detection and diagnosis of dental caries were done using CNNs for tooth classifications and diagnoses. Moreover, in this study, they aimed to evaluate the efficiency of deep CNNs because panoramic radiographs have different distortions according to the region being photographed [11].

Today, dental cavities usually occur due to the consumption of sugary drinks, food particles etc. When they are left in a tooth and some time passes, bacteria are generated. After this, plaque forms because of the mixed bacteria, saliva and acid. Soon after, the tooth enamel targets the plaque and results in the appearance of the familiar blackish holes. Hence, early diagnosis helps to avoid the development of dental illnesses, and the analysis of dental images allows for the accurate detection of dental disease in its early stages [8]. The method that Sukegawa et al. (2020) aimed to detect the early stages of cavities through Sobel Edge detection and deep CNN. Furthermore, contrast enhancement, histogram equalisation and feature selection were applied in the pre-processing stage. Additionally, diverse techniques of segmentation were used for comparison, namely Watershed and Otsu's threshold. The proposed method detected the edges in the dental images using the Sobel method and was applied in the gradient measurement of the intensity values of the pixel in the Gx and Gy directions. They concluded that the proposed method accomplished a 96.08% accuracy for its rate of prediction in comparison to other methods [8].

Notably, most oral lesions can develop into oral cancer. Moreover, the primary diagnosis of oral cancer involves examining the ocular regions accurately and recording the patient's oral cavity with true-colour digital images. Following this, the choice of further treatment for the patient with oral cancer mostly relies on the appearance of the lesion [9]. In Prabhakar and Rajaguru (2017), it was suggested that oral cancer is classified into two types: pathological and clinical. The goal was to assist the diagnosis of oral cancer patients using neural network classifiers. In the study, 75 oral cancer patients were examined with the help of Tumour Node Metastasis (TNM). The TNM variables were regarded as the input variables, and the results showed that the average accuracy of the classification was 100% for stage 1, 85.19% for stage 2, 84.21% for stage 3 and 94.12% for stage 4. Notably, the TNM accuracy results were compared to the linear layer neural network. Thus, these mentioned diagnostic tests can help to determine the stages of oral cancer, as well as help to make a treatment decision [9].

In the dental field, X-ray image techniques are classified into two categories: One technique is intraoral radiography, which is obtained from within the mouth of the patient, and the other technique is extraoral radiography, which is obtained from outside the mouth of the patient. In 2017, researchers proposed applying deep learning methods, such as tooth segmentation, to dental X-ray images depending on the detection and segmentation of every tooth in the panoramic images. Moreover, they used 1500 panoramic images in their study, even though it is considered a difficult way to isolate teeth through panoramic images because they show some parts of the patient's body, such as their jaw and chin, as well. Thus, the researchers suggested an automated method of segmentation for isolating. Consequently, this technique may be a start to assist dentists with their diagnoses through panoramic images [10].

In 2020, researchers in Japan performed a study on dental implants. They presented a classification model of various dental implant brands based on using the deep learning method. Moreover, it focused on using CNNs with panoramic X-rays for classification. Therefore, they applied and evaluated five models of CNN for implant classification.

However, among the five models, the finely tuned VGG16 model displayed the best performance in classifying implant brands in panoramic X-rays [12].

2.3 The Importance of Pulp Stone Detection

In dentistry, dental pulp is living tissue that survives due to the steady flow of blood. Pulp stones, often observed in bitewing and periapical radiographs, are separate calcified bodies in the dental pulp of healthy, diseased and unerupted teeth. Further, pulp stones vary in size, ranging from small, microscopic particles to large masses that almost occlude the pulp chamber. Additionally, they are more common in the coronal locations than in the pulp's radicular portions [13].

Memon et al. (2018), the authors conducted a study aiming to radiologically detect pulp stones and investigate any association between the occurrence of pulp stones and age, gender, the type of tooth, the dental arch and the status of the tooth. It was discovered that 21.7% of the patients suffering from renal stones had pulp stones and that a local or systematic pathology may increase the number or size of pulp stones. Hence, a correlation may exist between local or systemic pathologies and the occurrence of pulp stones. Moreover, the detection of vague objects is integral for the future of dental clinical support systems. In Fig. 1, two images from this research's dataset are displayed. The left side of the image shows a healthy tooth, while the right side of the image shows a tooth with a pulp stone.

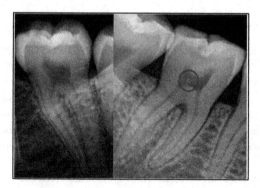

Fig. 1. A healthy tooth (left), and a tooth with a pulp stone (right).

3 Methodology

In the following section, we will discuss our methodology to detect and classify pulp stones. Figure 2 shows the framework for the proposed methodology.

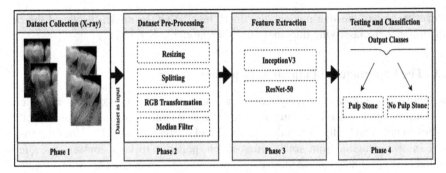

Fig. 2. Framework for the proposed methodology.

3.1 Dataset

The Information Technology department at Taibah University Dental Hospital in Al-Medina, KSA, archived and collected the dataset. A total of 212 periapical radiographs of female patients from 2019 to 2021 were selected and converted from RVG format to PNGs. Additionally, the dataset was divided into two folders: The first was labelled 'Stone' and contained 106 periapical radiographs showing pulp stones, and the other was labelled 'No Stone' and contained 106 periapical radiographs showing no pulp stones. The dataset was divided with the help of a radiology specialist.

3.2 The Pre-processing Stage

Since we aimed to classify X-ray images based on the detection of small and fine objects in the tooth pulp, CNN was chosen. The choice of CNN was mainly because of its capability to classify images, as well as its models' reduced computational time. Image pre-processing is a crucial technique that handles discrepancies and faults in images and prepares them for the upcoming procedures within the CNN models. Often, X-ray images contain some unclear boundaries and other defects such as poor exposure. In our case, we resized the dataset images for each model: The images were resized to 299 × 299 for the Inception v3 model and 224 × 224 for the Residual Network 50 (ResNet-50) model. The images were also converted from greyscale to RGB scale. Additionally, due to the targeting of fine and vague objects in the X-rays, we applied a median filter to remove the noise from the images. After that, the following techniques were applied to these pre-processed images.

3.3 Feature Extraction

In our method, we considered two different pre-trained CNN models, namely the Inception v3 and ResNet-50. The ResNet-50 was chosen because of its capability to handle complex problems while maintaining good performance, while the Inception v3 model was selected for its efficiency in detecting specific features that are inconsistent in size. To follow is a brief description of the models, along with their architecture.

ResNet-50: One of the known CNNs is the ResNet-50. It is a 50-layer deep model that was trained using a large number of images from the ImageNet database. The ResNet-50 can classify images into 1000 categories based on objects [22]. Additionally, the model contains five stages that are residual blocks, each of which contains layers and convolutions [20]. The overall architecture can be seen in Fig. 3.

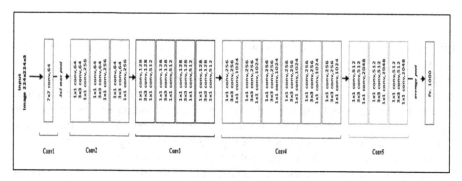

Fig. 3. The ResNet-50 [20].

Inception v3: Szegedy et al. first introduced the Inception v3 model in 2016. It is a CNN classification architecture that takes three convolutions with different window sizes and joins them all together [18]. Thus, the joining is done by chaining the three outputs into a single value. Then, the single-value output becomes the input of the next stage. Further, max pooling is connected with the convolution layers as an assessment additional to the classification process. Moreover, another 1×1 convolutional layer is added to the overall architecture. Hence, the overall architecture can be seen in Fig. 4.

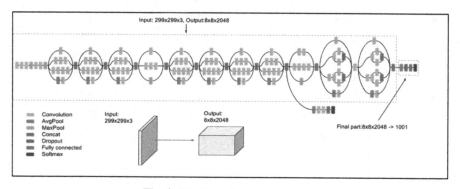

Fig. 4. The Inception v3 model [19].

3.4 The Classification Stage

After we extracted the features, the classification task was accomplished using different classifiers, namely the Support Vector Machine (SVM), Logistic Regression (LR) and K-Nearest Neighbours (KNN).

4 Experimentation

This section represents the experiments we performed to accomplish our goal of detecting pulp stones accurately. We used MATLAB (Ver 9.4.0) and uploaded our dataset to the MATLAB platform. The experiment consisted of two phases that differed in the size of their datasets but were identical in the rest of the processes. The dataset of the first phase contained 106 images in total, while the dataset of the second phase was expanded to 212 images. First, the dataset was randomly split into two sets: 70% for training and 30% for testing. Further pre-processing was performed, including resizing the images, transforming greyscale to RGB and applying the median filter to the dataset. Then, each of the two models, the Inception v3 [19] and ResNet-50 [7], was tested with the pre-processed dataset. By the end of the compilation, the feature labels, in addition to the testing and training, were extracted for each model. Furthermore, we evaluated the models' performance and applied different classifiers to each. In Table 1, the accuracy that the multiple classifiers of the two models obtained is listed.

Table 1. Obtained results from applying multiple classifiers to the pre-trained convolutional neural network models.

Phases	Classifier	Feature extractor	
		Inception v3	Resnet50
'One'	Cubic SVM	82.1%	81.1%
	Medium Gaussian SVM	81.1%	84%
	Logistic Regression	62.3%	58.5%
	Fine KNN	75.5%	78.3%
'Two'	Cubic SVM	72.6%	75.5%
	Medium Gaussian SVM	73.1%	76.4%
	Logistic Regression	51.4%	56.1%
	Fine KNN	67.5%	67%

5 Results and Discussion

In the experiment, we started with 106 images equally divided into stone and non-stone radiographs as our dataset. As a result, the ResNet-50 model reached an accuracy of 84% with the Medium Gaussian classifier, while the Inception v3 reached an accuracy of 81.1% with the same classifier. However, with the expansion of the dataset to reach a total of 212 images, it was noted that the accuracy of the two models decreased. In the second phase, the ResNet-50 reached an accuracy of 76.4% with the Medium Gaussian SVM classifier, while the Inception v3's accuracy with the same classifier was 73.1%. Notably, the ResNet-50 still excelled in comparison to the Inception v3 model. Ultimately, the accuracy results of the SVM classifiers for the two models were considered close. Figure 5 shows the results of the first phase, while Fig. 6 shows the results of the second phase.

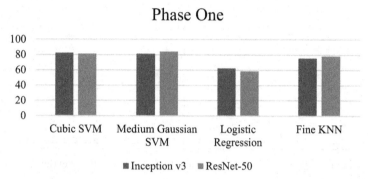

Fig. 5. A bar graph of the area under the curve obtained from applying multiple classifiers to the pre-trained convolutional neural network models—Phase one.

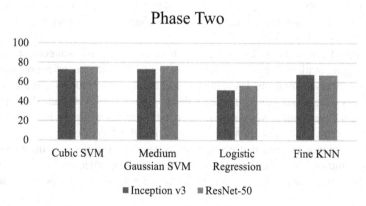

Fig. 6. A bar graph of the area under the curve obtained from applying multiple classifiers to the pre-trained convolutional neural network models—Phase two.

The area under the Receiver Operating Characteristic (ROC) curve summarised the performance of the two models after the use of multiple classifiers. We were interested in the ROC curve of the second phase since it represented a challenge due to its larger dataset. In Fig. 7, the ROC curve on the left side of the image shows that the ResNet-50 model incorrectly assigned 34% of the observations to the positive class. However, the model also correctly assigned 70% of the observations to the positive class. Overall, the total accuracy of the performance reached 0.70 for the ResNet-50 model. On the other hand, in Fig. 7, the ROC curve on the right side of the image shows that the Inception v3 model incorrectly assigned 41% and correctly assigned 58% of the observations to the positive class. Thus, the Inception v3 reached a total performance accuracy of 0.64.

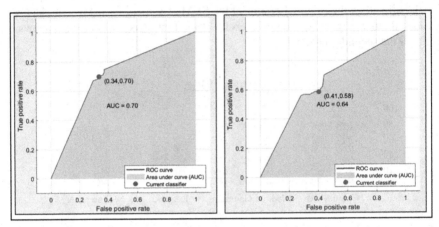

Fig. 7. The receiver operating characteristic curve for the ResNet-50 model (left), and Inception v3 model (Right).

Hence, these results suggest that the ResNet-50 is the best model for detecting pulp stones in radiographs since the false positive rate of the ResNet-50 was lower than that of the Inception v3, and the accuracy of the classifiers was better with the ResNet-50 than with the Inception v3.

It was noted that the flexibility of the chosen technique was advantageous because the parallel implementation of the different models from the same categories provided space for observation and alteration. Thus, the enhancements of the models and the choice of the classifiers were easier. However, the needed computational power and the complexity of the models were limited. Moreover, it was concluded that while the ResNet-50 model had the ability to classify pulp stones in radiographs, the decrease in accuracy when the dataset was expanded shows that it needs improvement. Additionally, the fuzziness of some of the radiographs, along with the vagueness of the object to be detected, made the classification more challenging and may have increased the false positive rate.

6 Conclusion

CNN usage in the medical field is increasing, and different applications are appearing every day. This paper aimed to assess the potential that CNN models have to detect fine and vague objects in dental radiographs. The fine objects we aimed to detect were pulp stones. Notably, pulp stones are objects that may be unclear for the observer to notice instantly, especially for dental students who are not yet used to the details of radiographs. We tested and compared the performance of two CNN models, namely the ResNet-50 and Inception v3, with multiple classifiers. The ResNet-50 model reached an accuracy of 76.4% with the Medium Gaussian SVM, while the Inception v3 reached an accuracy of 73.1% with the same classifier. Importantly, this experiment clarified the potential for uncovering the fine and vague details of dental radiographs accurately. It also clarified that the application of CNNs is promising in terms of uncovering the vague details of dental radiographs and can be used in clinical decision support systems.

7 Future Work

We aim to continue in the same domain and improve our methodology for detecting pulp stones in X-ray images. Further, we aim to increase the accuracy of our methodology by applying enhancements to the model architectures used.

Acknowledgements. The authors would like to express their appreciation to Dr Ebtihal H. Zain Alabdeen, assistant professor of oral radiology dentistry at the College of Dentistry at Taibah University for her great help and effort during the data preparation.

References

1. Karthick, K., Premkumar, M., Manikandan, R., Cristin, R.: Survey of image processing based applications in AMR. Rev. Comput. Eng. Res. **5**(1), 12–19 (2018)
2. Litjens, G., et al.: A survey on deep learning in medical image analysis. Med. Image Anal, **42**, 60–88 (2017)
3. Schwendicke, F., Golla, T., Dreher, M., Krois, J.: Convolutional neural networks for dental image diagnostics: a scoping review. J. Dent. **91**, 103226 (2019)
4. Soltanimehr, E., Bahrampour, E., Imani, M., Rahimi, F., Almasi, B., Moattari, M.: Effect of virtual versus traditional education on theoretical knowledge and reporting skills of dental students in radiographic interpretation of bony lesions of the jaw. BMC Med. Educ. **19**(1) (2019)
5. Ahn, E., Kumar, A., Kim, J., Li, C., Feng, D., Fulham, M.: X-ray image classification using domain transferred convolutional neural networks and local sparse spatial pyramid. In: IEEE 13th International Symposium on Biomedical Imaging (ISBI), pp. 855–858 (2016)
6. Privado, M., Villalón, J., Martínez, C., Ivorra, C.: Dental images recognition technology and applications: a literature review. Appl. Sci. **10**(8), 2856 (2020)
7. He, K., Zhang, X., Ren, S., Sun, J.: Deep residual learning for image recognition. In: Proceedings of the IEEE Conference on Computer Vision and Pattern Recognition, pp. 770–778 (2016)
8. Muthu Lakshmi, M., Chitra, P.: Classification of dental cavities from X-ray images using deep CNN algorithm. In: 4th International Conference on Trends in Electronics and Informatics (ICOEI) (48184), pp. 774–779 (2020)
9. Prabhakar, S., Rajaguru, H.: Performance analysis of linear layer neural networks for oral cancer classification. In: 6th ICT International Student Project Conference (ICT-ISPC), pp. 1–4 (2017)
10. Jader, G., Fontinele, J., Ruiz, M., Abdalla, K., Pithon, M., Oliveira, L.: Deep instance segmentation of teeth in panoramic X-ray images. In: 2018 31st SIBGRAPI Conference on Graphics, Patterns and Images (SIBGRAPI), IEEE, Parana (2018)

11. Lee, J.-H., Kim, D.-H., Jeong, S.-N., Choi, S.-H.: Detection and diagnosis of dental caries using a deep learning-based convolutional neural network algorithm. J. Dent. **77**, 106–111 (2018)

12. Sukegawa, S., et al.: Deep neural networks for dental implant system classification. Biomolecules **10** (2020)

13. Galav, A., Vyas, T., Kaur, M., Chauhan, M., Satija, N.: Association of pulp stones & renal stones- a clinical study. J. Oral. Biol. Craniofac. Res. **5**(3), 189–192 (2018)

14. Memon, M., Kalhoro, F.A., Shams, S., Arain, S.: A study on radiographic assessment of pulp stone. J. Endod. **25**, 992–996 (2018)

15. Khan, S., Yong, S.-P.: A Deep learning architecture for classifying medical images of anatomy object. In: 2017 Asia-Pacific Signal and Information Processing Association Annual Summit and Conference (APSIPA ASC). IEEE, Kuala Lumpur (2017)

16. oktay, A.B.: Tooth detection with convolutional neural networks. BioMed. Res. Int. **2021** (2017)

17. Szegedy, C., Vanhoucke, V., Ioffe, S., Shlens, J., Wojna, Z.: Rethinking the inception architecture for computer vision. In: 2016 IEEE Conference on Computer Vision and Pattern Recognition (CVPR) (2016)

18. Xia, X., Xu, C., Nan, B.: Inception-v3 for flower classification. In: 2017 2nd International Conference on Image, Vision and Computing (ICIVC) (2017)

19. Papers with code - Inception-v3 explained: Paperswithcode.com. https://paperswithcode.com/method/inception-v3. Accessed: 12 Dec 2020

20. Almabdy, S., Elrefaei, L.: Feature extraction and fusion for face recognition systems using pre-trained convolutional neural networks. Int. J. Comput. Digit. Syst. **9** (2020)

21. Rezende, E., Ruppert, G., Carvalho, T., Ramos, F., De Geus, P.: Malicious software classification using transfer learning of resnet-50 deep neural network. In: 2017 16th IEEE International Conference on Machine Learning and Applications (ICMLA), pp. 1011–1014. IEEE (2017)

22. Meghana, A.S., Sudhakar, S., Arumugam, G., Srinivasan, P., Prakash, K.B.: Age and gender prediction using convolution, ResNet50 and inception ResNetV2. Int. J. Adv. Trends Comput. Sci. Eng. **9** (2020)

Identification of Drug-Drug Interactions Using OCR

Enas Saleem Alrehily[(⊠)], Rawan Fahad Alhejaili, Dalal Rasheed Albeladi, and Liyakathunisa Syed

College of Computer Science and Engineering, Taibah University, Medinah, Saudi Arabia
ealrehily@outlook.sa, lansari@taibah.edu.sa

Abstract. Text detection and recognition in natural images have recently gained the attention of many researchers. It plays a significant role in different applications such as labels package identifications, and many blind assistance applications. OCR is widely used for this purpose. Precisely, for the drug label identification. It can be used to detect the Drug-Drug Interaction (DDI) which considers as one of the challenging tasks in public health safety. In this research, OCR is used to detect and extract the drug name from the drug boxes. Then the extracted drug name is used as input for the DDI identification process. The results of the proposed system are promising.

Keywords: OCR · Drug-drug interactions · Text detection · Drug label

1 Introduction

Text detection and recognition in natural images have recently gained the attention of many researchers due to their various practical applications. It plays a significant role in different applications such as label package identifications, plate number recognition, and many blind assistance applications [1]. Optical Character Recognition (OCR) is widely used to detect and extract text from documents or images and convert it into a digital data format [2]. Recently, many researchers used OCR to detect and extract the drug label [2, 3].

However, text detection and recognition for drug packages can be beneficial for many applications e.g. drug tracking, dose controlling and drug prescription. Moreover, the drug name is a unique feature that distinguishes each drug from another [3]. It can be used to detect the Drug-Drug Interaction (DDI) which is considered as one of the challenging tasks in public health safety [4]. In this research, OCR is used to detect the drug name from natural drug images. The extracted name then will be used as input for the DDI identification process. Many papers have discussed different text detection issues. However, a few of them have discussed text detection and recognition in natural drug images. This paper is organized as follows. Section 2 present different recent drug recognition systems. Section 3 proposes Drug-Drug interactions identification systems. Experimental Results and Discussion in Sect. 4. Section 5 conclude the finding of the research in addition to future works.

© ICST Institute for Computer Sciences, Social Informatics and Telecommunications Engineering 2022
Published by Springer Nature Switzerland AG 2022. All Rights Reserved
S. Spinsante et al. (Eds.): HealthyIoT 2021, LNICST 432, pp. 125–135, 2022.
https://doi.org/10.1007/978-3-030-99197-5_11

2   Related Works

2.1   Drug Label Identification Through Image and Text Embedding Model

Liu et al. [2] developed a model called "Drug Label Identification through Image and Text embedding model (DLI-IT)" to detect suspicious drugs. First, they cropped the raw images into sub-images based on the text by training a Connectionist Text Proposal Network (CTPN). Then, they used the Tesseract OCR Engine to independently recognize the sub-images and combined them as one document for each row image. Finally, they transformed these documents into vectors by applying universal sentence embedding. Furthermore, they used the cosine similarity to find the similarity between the reference image and the test image. They showed that their model achieved up to 88% precision in drug label identification.

2.2   ST-Med-Box

Wan-Jung et al. [5] develop an intelligent medicine recognition system named "ST-Med-Box" to help chronic patients in organizing several medications they take to avoid drug interactions. Moreover, it gives users other functionalities related to medication like reminders of time to take medications, and some information about medication, as well as chronic patient information management. Authors need four things to build their system, an intelligent medicine recognition device, an application running on the Android platform, "Google TensorFlow" deep learning framework, and a cloud-based management platform. Their proposed system achieves an accuracy of up to 96.6%, so it is very effective in reducing drug interactions. Figure 1 illustrated their system.

Although the system has achieved high accuracy, it remains limited to chronic patients drugs so, it needs modifications so that it can be used on different types of drugs to discover interactions between them.

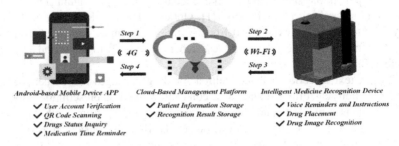

Fig. 1. "ST-Med-Box" system [5]

2.3   LSTM-CRF

Authors in [6] proposed the LSTM-CRF method based on a neural network to achieve the purpose of the Drug-Named Entity Recognition without the need for extra knowledge. This method takes the sequence of word embedding and character-level embedding from a sentence as an input vector and output a label sequence. However, they use two datasets, the DDI2011 and the DDI2013 and achieve precision rate up to 93.26%.

2.4 Syntax Convolutional Neural Network (SCNN)

Authors in [7] describe "syntax convolutional neural network (SCNN)" based DDI extraction approach. They also used word embedding (both syntax word embedding and novel word embedding) to declare the syntactic information of a sentence after that by using POS features, they recognize the POS data and the position. Experimental results of the proposed method achieve an F-score of 0.686.

However, the two related methods mentioned above are used a neural network to recognize drug name not interactions, but in the same field.

2.5 Position-Aware Deep Multi-task Learning Approach for Extracting DDIs from Biomedical Texts

Authors in [8] proposed a "position-aware deep multi-task learning approach for extracting DDIs from biomedical texts" to predict if two drugs will interact with each other or not. They also focus their approach on word and position embeddings. Also, they used (BiLSTM) network to encode every sentence. The proposed approach was applied to the "DDIExtraction challenge 2013 corpus" and achieves an F-score of 72.99%, so it considers an effective approach.

2.6 Recognition Medicine Name from Doctor's Prescription

Dhande et al. [9] proposed a method for recognition medicine name from doctor's prescription, this prescription is cursive English handwriting. The authors collected the data by scanning the document or taking a photo. The recognition achieved by three techniques, horizontal projection for text-line segmentation while vertical projection histogram for word segmentation. Lastly, SVM is applied for classification. The system produced fine results with total accuracy of 85%.

2.7 DDIs from Structured Product Labels

Tran et al. [10] proposed a method for detecting DDIs from structured product labels with linkage to standard terminologies by applying Deep learning architecture. Additionally, this framework detects the outcome of the interaction. Despite, there were 22 drug labels, 22 drug labels were used for training, additional 180 annotated drug labels have been utilized. Two test sets have been used they achieve 21.59% and 23.55% on relation extraction respectively. The result is not satisfactory enough the method need to be tested more to ensure its accuracy.

2.8 The Automated Drug Detection and Location Identification

Roy et al. [11] proposed a system aimed at serving blind people to identify and locate the drugs around them, whether it is mentioned in a picture or real-time video, via voice commands. To identify the name of the drug, they initially used Aspose optical character recognition tool but the error rate in it was high, around 37.2, so they moved to try the Google Tesseract tool and they obtained good results from it, the error rate did not exceed 25.4, so it was adopted in their proposed system. Moreover, for taking a frame from the video to extract characters and identify the name the proposed system used a Kinect sensor which worked effectively. Figure 2 below shows the block diagram for the system.

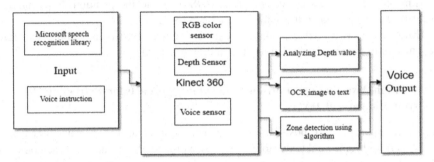

Fig. 2. The automated drug detection and location identification for visually impaired using image processing and voice commands system [11]

2.9 Drug-Drug Interaction Extraction

Demner-Fushman et al. [12] review the Text Analysis Conference (TAC 2018) Drug-Drug Interaction Extraction. Where the teams participating in the conference were given a pre-defined group of drug-drug interactions on a dataset contains 325 Product Labels and they were asked to fulfill four conditions: extracting drug interactions at the level of sentences, then identifying the substances interacting with each other, dividing these interactions and defining the group of distinct interactions in all given drugs. The teams' results were not sufficiently accurate and satisfactory, so more research was encouraged in the field of drug-drug interaction.

2.10 A Label Propagation Method with Linear Neighborhood Information

Zhang et al. [13] proposed a method called "a label propagation method with linear neighborhood information (LPLNI)" based on machine learning to predict drug-target interaction with linear neighborhood information. They evaluated and experimented with the method on four benchmark datasets produced by Yamanishi et al. [14] with pre-defined interaction and then try to predicate unknown ones. To ensure the correctness of predicted drug interactions, they check with the "SuperTarget" which is a database consisting of many drug interactions, they conclude that the proposed method can predict new interactions effectively and with high accuracy.

Table 1 summarizes the related works. Our main requirement is to reflect drug-drug interactions effectively using OCR. The overview represented above on the field of research showed that different types of proposed methods and systems can achieve high precision in drug label identification, but none of them applied OCR to identify drug-drug interaction which leads us to applied it to our proposed system due to its simplicity and fast scanning.

Table 1. Related works summary

Ref	Data used	Techniques	Accuracy
Liu et al. [2]	Samples from Daily-Med website	Partial Levenshtein Distance (PLD) and Tesseract OCR Engine	Up-to 88%
Wan-Jung et al. [5]	chronic patients drugs	"Google TensorFlow", and a cloud-based management platform	Up to 96.6%
Zeng et al. [6]	Two datasets, the DDI2011 and the DDI2013	LSTM-CRF method based on a neural network	Up to 93.26%
Zhao et al. [7]	-	Word embedding using POS features	Achieve an F-score of 0.686
Miao et al. [8]	The proposed approach was applied to the "DDI Extraction challenge 2013 corpus"	Word and position embeddings using (BiLSTM) network	Achieves an F-score of 72.99%
Dhande et al. [9]	Data collected by scanning the document or taking a photo	Horizontal projection, vertical projection histogram and SVM	Up to 85%
Tran et al. [10]	Two different test sets	Deep learning architecture	21.59% and 23.55%
Roy et al. [11]	Frames from real-time video	Google Tesseract tool and Kinect sensor	Error rate up to 25.4
Demner-Fushman et al. [12]	Dataset given by (TAC 2018) Conference	-	Results were not accurate
Zhang et al. [13]	Dataset produced by Yamanishi et al. [14]	(LPLNI) method based on machine learning	High accuracy

3   Methodology

Text detection and recognition using OCR has been used by many researchers for different purpose. In this research, we used OCR to detect and extract text from natural drugs images. This research proposed a system that utilizes OCR tool to detect and recognize drugs names from natural pictures taken by the authors. The following sections describe the dataset that used in this research and the proposed system.

3.1   Dataset

This section presents the dataset that utilized in this research. The dataset consists of 27 drug images collected from different websites based on the active ingredients of each drug. The interactions between the drugs is identified based on the data collected from 'Pharmacy Time' [15] as shown below:

- Fluoxetine interacts with Phenelzine
- Digoxin interacts with Quinidine
- Sildenafil interacts with Isosorbide Mononitrate
- Clonidine interacts with Propranolol
- Warfarin interacts with Diflunisal
- Theophylline interacts with Ciprofloxacin
- Methotrexate interacts with Probenecid
- Bromocriptine interacts with Pseudoephedrine

The interaction between drugs is identified based on this list. When a drug name is extracted and recognized by OCR, the system will search for a match. Precisely, each drug has different brand names. Thus, the system will search for the active ingredient or the brand name. For this reason, we linked each active ingredients with the corresponding brand names as shown in Table 2. The brand names of different drugs were taken from National Library of Medicine (NLM) website [16].

Table 2. Some of the active ingredients with their brand names.

Active ingredient	Brand name	Active ingredient	Brand name
Fluoxetine	Prozac, Rapiflux, Selfemra, Prozac Weekly, Sarafem	Phenelzine	Nardil
Digoxin	Cardoxin, Digitek, Lanoxicaps, Lanoxin	Quinidine	Cardioquin, CinQuin, Duraquin, Quinact,Quinaglute, Quinalan, Quinatime,
Sildenafil	Revatio, Viagra	Isosorbide Mononitrate	BiDil
Clonidine	Catapres, Jenloga, Kapvay	Propranolol	Inderal, InnoPran, Pronol
Warfarin	Coumadin, Jantoven	Diflunisal	Dolobid

3.2 The Proposed System

As the system need an image search, it used a simple technique with a ready function code for text recognition by optical character recognition (OCR). We used a function from Computer Vision Toolbox at MATLAB R2021a. The proposed model works as follows:

First, different preprocessing steps were applied on the images to increase the accuracy of the detection process, such as maximizing the image size and dealing with the drug name as a block instead of single characters [17]. After that, the drug image is input into the OCR code to extract the drug name. This OCR code is from then the extracted drug name goes through the DDI detection step. In the DDI detection step, a MATLAB code is used to search for a match between the extracted drug name and the drug names stored in the system. It ignored the case of the letters at drug name. If a match is found, drug interaction information will be displayed to the user. Otherwise, the system will display "no interaction is found!" as shown in Fig. 3. Figures 4 and 5 show the proposed system.

```
if (contains([ocrResults.Text],"Fluoxetine", 'IgnoreCase', true)||contains([ocrResults.Text],"Prozac", 'IgnoreCase',true))
 disp("Drug interaction: Phenelzine or Nardil ") ;
elseif (contains([ocrResults.Text],"Phenelzine",'IgnoreCase', true)||contains([ocrResults.Text],"Nardil",'IgnoreCase', true))
   disp("Drug interaction: Fluoxetine or Prozac") ;

 elseif (contains([ocrResults.Text], "Digoxin",'IgnoreCase', true) ||contains([ocrResults.Text],"Cardoxin",'IgnoreCase', true))
 disp("Drug interaction: Quinidine ") ;
elseif (contains([ocrResults.Text],"Quinidine",'IgnoreCase', true))
   disp("Drug interaction: Digoxin or Nardil ");

  elseif (contains([ocrResults.Text],"Sildenafil",'IgnoreCase', true) || contains([ocrResults.Text],"Revatio",'IgnoreCase', true))
  disp("Drug interaction: Isosorbide Mononitrate or BiDil") ;
elseif (contains([ocrResults.Text], "Isosorbide Mononitrate",'IgnoreCase', true )|| contains([ocrResults.Text],"BiDil",'IgnoreCase', true))
   disp("Drug interaction: Sildenafil or Revatio ") ;

elseif (contains([ocrResults.Text], "Clonidine",'IgnoreCase', true) || contains([ocrResults.Text], "Catapres",'IgnoreCase', true))
 disp("Drug interaction: Propranolol or Inderal") ;
elseif (contains([ocrResults.Text], "Propranolol",'IgnoreCase', true) ||contains([ocrResults.Text]," Inderal",'IgnoreCase', true))
   disp("Drug interaction: Clonidine or Catapres") ;

elseif (contains([ocrResults.Text], "Warfarin",'IgnoreCase', true )|| contains([ocrResults.Text]," Coumadin",'IgnoreCase', true))
 disp("Drug interaction: Diflunisal or Dolobid") ;
elseif (contains([ocrResults.Text],"Diflunisal",'IgnoreCase', true )|| contains([ocrResults.Text],"Dolobid",'IgnoreCase', true))
   disp("Drug interaction: Warfarin or Coumadin") ;

elseif (contains([ocrResults.Text],"Theophylline",'IgnoreCase',true))
 disp("Drug interaction: Ciprofloxacin") ;
elseif (contains([ocrResults.Text],"Ciprofloxacin",'IgnoreCase',true))
   disp("Drug interaction: Theophylline") ;

elseif (contains([ocrResults.Text],"Methotrexate",'IgnoreCase',true))
 disp("Drug interaction: Probenecid") ;
elseif(contains([ocrResults.Text],"Probenecid",'IgnoreCase',true))
   disp("Drug interaction: Methotrexate") ;

elseif (contains([ocrResults.Text],"Bromocriptine",'IgnoreCase',true))
 disp("Drug interaction: Pseudoephedrine") ;
elseif (contains([ocrResults.Text],"Pseudoephedrine",'IgnoreCase',true))
   disp("Drug interaction: Bromocriptine") ;

% If no interactions is found
else
   disp("No Drug interaction is Found") ;
end
```

Fig. 3. MATLAB code

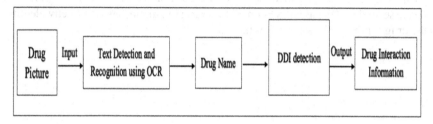

Fig. 4. The General architecture of the proposed system

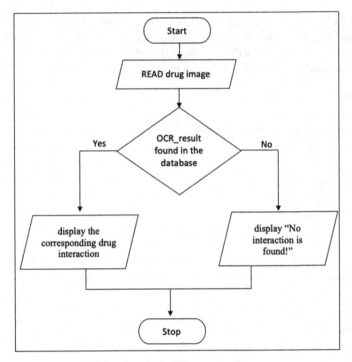

Fig. 5. Flowchart of the proposed system

4 Results and Discussion

The proposed system was tested on 27 drug images. We performed the proposed system on two different datasets. The first datasets consist of raw images without any preprocessing. For the second dataset, we performed different preprocessing steps on the images such as maximizing the image size and dealing with the drug name as a block instead of single characters [17].

However, the system failed to identify ten images when was tested for the first dataset. This false detection is due to different reasons such as font text type, the drug box shape (cylinder drug box is harder to detect) and inappropriate lighting (reflection of the light on the drug image) as shown in Table 3. The accuracy of the proposed system was 63%, while the second part the identification of drug-drug interactions was correctly identified all the drugs. Table 4 shows some of the results.

Table 3. False detection results of the proposed system

Drug	Preprocessing	OCR Results	Reasons
	Increase the image size	|NDERAI.'	Font text type
	Increase the length of the image	Jflunisal	Drug box shape is cylinder.
	Treat the text in the image as a single block of text and increase the image size	Dolol	Drug box shape is cylinder
	Increase the image size	Not recognized	Reflection of the light on the drug image
	Treats the text in the image as a single block of text	ugnldine Gluconate	Drug box shape is cylinder

Table 4. Some results of the proposed system

Drug	OCR Results	Drug-Interaction
	Ciprofloxacin	Theophylline
	PROZAC	Phenelzine or Nardil
	Probenecid	Methotrexate
	Bromocriptine	Pseudoephedrine
	Wartafm	Failed
	COUMHDiN	Failed

5   Conclusion

Nowadays, there are a lot of people around the world who suffer from different diseases and have to take several drugs together at the same time. In this research, a simple approach of DDI identification based on OCR is presented. In this approach drug pictures are taken as an input then the drug interaction information will display as the output. In the future, we aim to perform more training on the OCR using deep learning techniques to increase the accuracy. Also, we hope to develop our system so that it includes an audio reading to help the blind to identify their medications.

References

1. Kulkarni, C.R., Barbadekar, A.B.: Text detection and recognition: a review. Int. Res. J. Eng. Technol. **4**, 179–185 (2017)
2. Liu, X., Meehan, J., Tong, W., et al.: DLI-IT: a deep learning approach to drug label identification through image and text embedding. BMC Med. Inform. Decis. Mak. **20**, 1–9 (2020). https://doi.org/10.1186/s12911-020-1078-3
3. Nadarajan, A.S., Thamizharasi, A.: A survey on text detection in natural images. Int. J. Eng. Dev. Res. **6**(1), 60–66 (2018)
4. Ribeiro, B., Alves, N., Guevara, M, Magalhães, L.; A three-staged approach to medicine box recognition. In: EPCGI 2017 - 24th Encontro Port Comput Graf e Interacao 2017-Janua 1–7 (2017). https://doi.org/10.1109/EPCGI.2017.8124317
5. Chang, W.J., Chen, L.B., Hsu, C.H., Lin, C.P., Yang, T.C.: A deep learning-based intelligent medicine recognition system for chronic patients. IEEE Access **7**. 44441–44458 (2019)
6. Zeng, D., Sun, C., Lin, L., Liu, B.: LSTM-CRF for drug-named entity recognition. Entropy **19**(6), 283 (2017)
7. Zhao, Z., Yang, Z., Luo, L., Lin, H., Wang, J.: Drug-drug interaction extraction from biomedical literature using syntax convolutional neural network. Bioinformatics **32**, 3444–3453,)2016(
8. Zhou, D., Miao, M., He, Y.: Position-aware deep multi-task learning for drug–drug interaction extraction. Artif. Intell. Med. **87**, 1–8 (2018)
9. Dhande, P.S., Kharat, R.: Character recognition for cursive english handwriting to recognize medicine name from doctor's prescription. In: 2017 International Conference on Computing, Communication, Control and Automation (ICCUBEA), pp. 1–5, August 2017
10. Tran, T., Kavuluru, R., Kilicoglu, H.: A Multi-task learning framework for extracting drugs and their interactions from drug labels. arXiv preprint arXiv:1905.07464 (2019)
11. Roy, U., Alam, M.A.: Automated drug detection and location identification for visually impaired using image processing and voice commands (2017)
12. Demner-Fushman, D., Fung, K.W., Do, P., Boyce, R.D., Goodwin, T.R.: Overview of the TAC 2018 drug-drug interaction extraction from drug labels track. In: Proceedings of the Text Analysis Conference (TAC) 2018, Gaithersburg, 13–14 November 2018 (2019)
13. Zhang, W., Chen, Y., Li, D.: Drug-target interaction prediction through label propagation with linear neighborhood information. Molecules **22**(12), 1–14 (2017)
14. Yamanishi, Y., Araki, M., Gutteridge, A., Honda, W., Kanehisa, M.: Prediction of drug-target interaction networks from the integration of chemical and genomic spaces. Bioinformatics **24**(13), 232–240 (2008)
15. 2002-10-6975 @ www.pharmacytimes.com. https://www.pharmacytimes.com/publications/issue/2002/2002-10/2002-10-6975. Accessed 21 Jan 2021
16. National Library of Medicine - National Institutes of Health. In: Nlm.nih.gov. https://www.nlm.nih.gov/. Accessed 22 Feb 2021
17. MathWorks: ocr. https://www.mathworks.com/help/vision/ref/ocr.html. Accessed 21 Jan 2021

Applied Computing - Physical Sciences and Engineering

Patients Behaviour Monitoring Inside a Hospital Garden: Comparison Between RADAR and GPS Solutions

Gianluca Ciattaglia[✉][ID], Deivis Disha[ID], Adelmo De Santis[ID], and Ennio Gambi[ID]

Università Politecnica delle Marche, Via Brecce Bianche, 60131 Ancona, Italy
{g.ciattaglia,d.disha}@pm.univpm.it, {adelmo.desantis,e.gambi}@univpm.it

Abstract. Monitoring the behaviors of inpatients with reduced cognitive abilities within an area of a hospital can provide important information on how patients live in that space and which part is of most interest. In this paper two different techniques are applied to perform this monitoring in an outdoor space; the former is based on the GPS positioning and timing, and the subjects must wear a suitable device, while the latter is based on a non-contact radar technology. Radar sensors are in fact nowadays very powerful even for medical applications and can be used to monitor patients within environments. In this work, the behaviors monitoring of the people inside the garden of a retirement house is considered. The two different techniques are used for tracking the subjects and the results are compared.

Keywords: GPS · AAL · Tracking · Radar · Smartwatch

1 Introduction

The availability of automotive radars, introduced to improve vehicle safety, has made it possible to have very reliable radar systems at a relatively low cost. As required by the standard they transmit with a carrier frequency of around 80 GHz, and to provide high performances the transmission bandwidth is very large [11,17]. These systems are powerful not only in the automotive field but can be also applied for improving the safety of the living environment, where the detection of people and the prediction of any dangerous situations represents another classical problem that can be solved with radars [1,13]. Thanks to the performance of the modern mmWave automotive radars, it is possible to track a person inside an ambient with a very good resolution [8]. Another key point on the usage of these systems for Ambient Assisted Living (AAL) is the capability offered by the Multiple In Multiple Out (MIMO) technology. With MIMO radars non only the distance can be detected, but also the angular position of a target, through the evaluation in a very fast way of the Angle of Arrival (AoA) without moving the sensor [12]. Modern four-dimensional MIMO automotive radar

S. Spinsante et al. (Eds.): HealthyIoT 2021, LNICST 432, pp. 139–152, 2022.
https://doi.org/10.1007/978-3-030-99197-5_12

provides a very high angular resolution, as in the automotive field AoA information is crucial for autonomous driving. The performance of typical automotive radars makes them interesting in the AAL context to track people within the living environment and obtain information on their behavior through suitable processing of the radar signal.

Monitoring the activity of a person can be done also with other radio technology, for example in [16,18] an approach based on Long Range (LoRa) communication is proposed. In these cases, a specific device must be suited by the patient, and also the area of usage must be covered by the LoRa access points. Another approach to solving the problem of tracking people is to use a smartwatch equipped with GPS. The usage of a smartwatch for healthcare applications is very common as the device integrates many sensors that can be used for monitoring the conditions of a patient. In [14], a smartwatch is used to monitor a patient affected by dementia, and in [3] the GPS is used to collect information about Schizophrenic Patients. With this device the tracking of a person inside an area is simple to implement but, since the smartwatch needs to receive the GPS satellite signal to obtain its position, its operation is precluded indoor, or where the signals of satellites cannot be received. On the other hand, smartwatches equipped with GPS receivers are very popular and relatively low cost and allow a relatively accurate definition of the position.

In this work, the two different approaches are applied to study the movements of people within an outdoor environment, the garden of a retirement home. In this garden, areas of sensory stimulation have been created, through flowerbeds with colored flowers, aromatic plants, and the diffusion of music. This work aims to propose a technological tool that can objectively define which of these areas attract the attention of patients with reduced cognitive abilities, and how long patients stay within these areas. The paper describes the technologies used, and the results obtained are shown and compared, highlighting the strengths and weaknesses of the two proposed technologies.

2   The Considered Technologies

2.1   Radar Systems

The radars used in this work are two 4D imaging radars, that are designed for Advanced Driver-Assistance Systems (ADAS) applications. They implement the Frequency Modulated Continuous Wave (FMCW) scheme and the MIMO technology. The transmitted signal ranges from 77 GHz to a maximum of 81 GHz and the bandwidth may reach the value of 4 GHz. Each radar board is composed of four single-chip radar, each of one is characterized by four receivers and three transmitters antennas. The position of all the antennas provides a very high resolution along the azimuth plane, but it is also possible to detect the elevation of the targets [6]. These devices are the new frontier in ADAS as their capabilities to track and classify the target type are very promising [9,15]. In this work, only the position along the azimuth plane is of interest, and the data collected by the elevation elements of the antenna array are neglected.

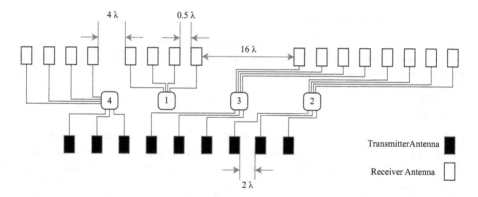

Fig. 1. MIMO antennas layout for improving AoA resolution along the azimuth plane.

A description of the transmitter and receiver antennas is shown in Fig. 1, where the horizontal distance between the antennas connected to the same chip and between the antennas connected to the four chips are highlighted. In Fig. 1, λ is the wavelength of the transmitted signal. The positions of the antennas are fundamental to realizing the virtual array used in this work and this is obtained by performing a spatial convolution between the transmitter and the receivers antennas. Considering only the transmitters indicated in Fig. 1, the result is a planar array of 86 elements along the azimuth plane. To avoid the overlapping of the signals transmitted, different channel access schemes can be assigned to the two radar boards, the Time Division Multiplexing and the Binary Phase Modulation [10]. For simplicity and to avoid any phase imperfection the first one is chosen, so each transmitted chirp is sent by following the order configured inside the device. The transmitted chirps are grouped inside a frame and at least one chirp for each transmitter must be sent. In the FMCW scheme, at the receiver side, the transmitted and the received signals are mixed and the result is another signal called beat signal, which is sampled by an analog to digital converter. The higher the frequency of the beat signal, the greater the distance to the target that reflected the radar signal. The maximum detectable range R_{max} is related to the maximum beat frequency according to the equation:

$$R_{max} = \frac{c \cdot f_b}{2 \cdot S} \tag{1}$$

where c is the speed of light, f_b the beat frequency and S the chirp ramp slope [7]. Since the maximum detectable beat rate is related to the sample rate, increasing it allows a higher range to be detected. All the collected data are stored inside a Solid State Drive (SSD) that is directly connected to the radar board. For each device, the collected samples of the beat signals are stored inside a raw file that contains the complex values of each sample.

2.2   Smartwatch with GPS

Most of the modern smartwatches are equipped with GPS and these devices are the simplest way to detect their position. In this work two models of smartwatches are considered:

- Garmin Fenix 6
- Garmin VivoActive 4

Both the models are designed to support the user during a training session, and can provide information from different on board sensors about: user location, altitude, speed, and GPS accuracy; or about user activity such as heart rate or acceleration.

The devices can record all the sensors' data by using an appropriate application called "RawLogger" and a custom Python script was developed to save them on a computer. The data are not directly exported in a human-readable format, so the script can extract the data and store them inside a Comma Separated Value (CSV) file. For each row, the file contains a sample of each sensor and the samples are marked with a progressive time-stamp. In this case, only the GPS data are considered as only the position of the user is of interest for this work.

GPS data can be processed not only with the custom developed software but also through the cloud platform provided by GARMIN, the vendor of the devices. In Fig. 2 the results of the two processing methods are compared. Data are acquired by Fenix 6, and the blue and red line represent the results of custom and cloud methods respectively. From the figure it is possible to see how both methods provide very similar results, the curves being almost perfectly overlapping. On the contrary in Fig. 3 a comparison between the accuracy of two smartwatches worn by the same person can be found. In the figure, red line shows the result obtained with Fenix 6, while blue line the one obtained with VivoActive 4.

The different paths represented in the figure are the result of the different hardware inside the smartwatches, which are characterized by a different precision. It is also necessary to take into account the different number of satellites that each smartwatch can receive, since this leads to a different precision.

3   Measurement Setup and Radar Signal Processing

3.1   Measurement Area and Systems Configuration

The measurement area is a garden of a retirement home whose plan can be found in Fig. 4a. Inside the garden are present trees, metal chairs and other stuff such as a gazebo and a small pool. The green lines in the figure represent walls and the grey line near the perimeter trees is a metal fence. From Fig. 4b the presence of the trees and walls is highlighted. As the purpose of this work is to identify and track the position of the people inside the garden all these objects contribute, through the global clutter produced by the environment on the radar signal, to a decrease in the accuracy of the position.

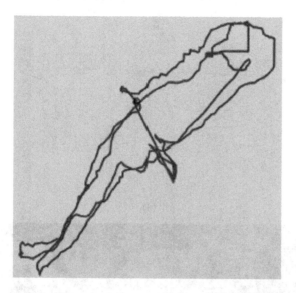

Fig. 2. Comparison between the custom processing and the cloud processing (Color figure online)

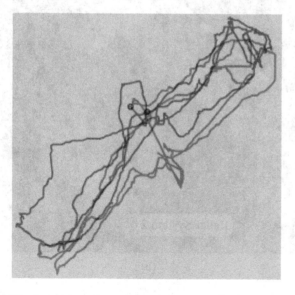

Fig. 3. GPS positioning detection comparison with the two different smartwatches. (Color figure online)

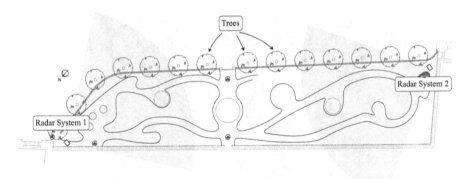

(a)

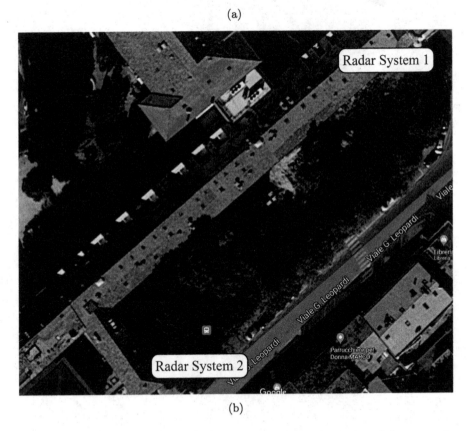

(b)

Fig. 4. Measurement setup area: a) plan of the garden and position of the two radar systems; b) picture from the satellite of the same area. (Color figure online)

The longest sides of the garden are about equal to 90 m and the shortest 25 m. The two radar systems, whose positions are shown in the figure, are configured with the same parameters so to avoid mutual interference. The configuration parameters can be found in Table 1.

Table 1. Radar configuration parameters.

Parameter	Value
Start frequency [GHz]	77
Chirp slope [MHz/μs]	49.97
Idle time [μs]	5
ADC start time [μs]	6
Ramp end time [μs]	80
ADC sampling rate [MHz]	10
Number of samples per chirp	512
Chirps per frame	12
Inter-frame interval [ms]	1000

The description of the parameters follows:

- Start Frequency: carrier start frequency, with this system the carrier goes from 77 to a maximum of 81 GHz;
- Chirp Slope: Slope of the chirp frequency, a high slope can produce a chirp with a bigger bandwidth in less time;
- Idle time: idle time between two chirps, this time is used to restore the ramp generator inside the device;
- Ramp end Time: time length of the transmitted chirp;
- ADC Sampling Rate: sampling rate of the beat signal at each receiver;
- ADC start time: the chirp frequency is controlled by a ramp generator, in the first part the ramp is not linear so this time is used to neglect this samples;
- Number of samples per chirp: the number of samples used in each chirp;
- Chirps per frame: as described before the transmitted chirps are grouped in frames;
- Inter-frame Interval: each frame has a certain duration, this time is always less than Ramp end Time × Chirps per frame.

With the configuration of Table 1, the maximum detectable range is around 30 m so the two radar systems can detect less than half of the garden area. The choice of this configuration is related to the aperture of the antenna system and the reduction of the range capability can decrease the amount of undesired clutter. The Inter-Frame Interval is chosen equal to one second, in order to limit the total amount of data produced by the system. As the observed targets are moving slowly inside the area, the beat signal, and then the spatial data, can be sampled at a slow rate.

To perform the measurements with the GPS each person wears the Fenix 6 on the left arm and the VivoActive 4 on the right arm. The GPS data are collected by the two devices and processed in both the ways, cloud and custom.

3.2 Radar Signal Processing

The samples of each beat signal are taken from each data file and reorganized in a five-dimensional data-cube, are then stored following this method:

- The samples of each chirp are the fast-time samples and these samples are stored along with the rows of a matrix, each column of this matrix contains the samples of each transmitted chirp and are called slow-time;
- For each transmitted chirp, the reflected signal is received by all the elements of the virtual array so along two other dimensions the samples related to the azimuth and the elevation plane are stored;
- As this four-dimensional hyper-cube is generated for each frame the fifth dimension is the time evolution of the acquisition.

Once the five-dimensional data-cube was built the range-azimuth maps are evaluated, since the main purpose of the radar system is to track the position of the people inside the area. The maps are obtained by performing a bi-dimensional Fast Fourier Transform on the plane fast-time - azimuth. The result is a cube where each "slice" is a range-azimuth map. In each range-azimuth map, a two-dimensional Constant False Alarm Rate (CFAR) [8] detector is applied, in order to reduce most of noise and clutter. The environment where the measurements are performed is very dense and trees, lightning lights, and big flowerpots are present; the 2D-CFAR provides a more clear view of the maps obtained from the radar. An example of the obtained result is depicted in Fig. 5a.

The threshold calculated by the 2D-CFAR changes according to the elements around the Cell Under Test (CUT) so the threshold is adaptive along with the map and in this way the clutter is reduced. Only the CUTs where the intensity value is over the threshold are revealed. The values of the final map are zero or one according to whether the threshold has been exceeded or not. The application of the 2D-CFAR threshold provides the positions of the possible targets; when they occupy more CUTs by applying the DBSCAN technique [5] the points are grouped and a single target is revealed. The best performance for this algorithm is provided from a DBSCAN with a square-euclidean distance of ten and the minimum number of points that compose a target equal to five. An example result can be found in Fig. 5b.

With the aim to study the movements of the people inside the garden it is necessary to remove the background, due to the signal reflected by the static objects. These are elements inside the DBSCAN result maps and to remove them the Mixture of Gaussian (MoG) algorithm is applied [2]. The result of MoG applied to the maps after the DBSCAN is depicted inside Fig. 6.

After retrieving all the maps using the background Subtraction algorithm the Tracker Video Analysis and Modeling tool is used for tracking the movement of the people inside the observed area [4].

4 Experimental Tests and Results

In order to test and compare the different acquisition systems, four different tests were performed:

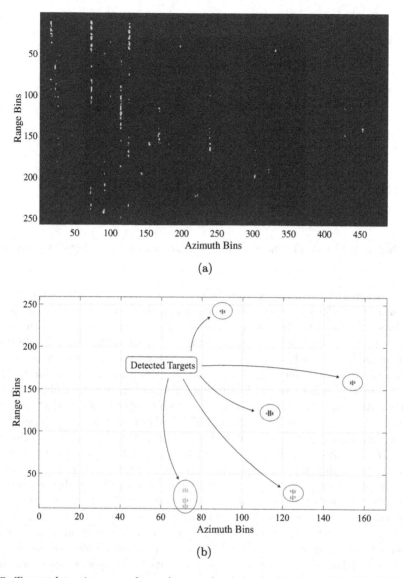

Fig. 5. Target detection procedure: a) example of the application of the 2D-CFAR on the Range-Azimuth map; b) resulting map after the DBSCAN application.

- two thirty-minute acquisitions with many people involved;
- a ten-minute acquisition with only two people involved;
- a five-minute acquisition with only two people involved;

The position of the radars are chosen properly to obtain as much information from the individual people that were doing different activities like walking, sitting on chair, and others. In Fig. 7 the path of one subject during all the time of the

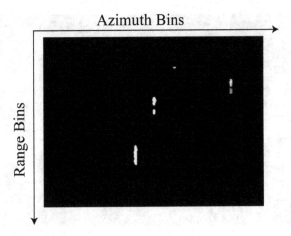

Fig. 6. Application of the MoG background removal to the DBSCAN maps.

measurement is shown, as received by each radar. Since the detection range of the radar is smaller than the size of the garden, the final image of the trajectory is obtained by merging the data from both radars. The radar acquisitions started at the same time and have the same duration. In this time the subjects moved from the area covered by one radar to the other one. During the measurements different targets are observed and the main problem is related to the impossibility with the proposed method to identify the targets when moving from one area to another. An exact evaluation requires the presence of only one subject moving at a time; when two or more subjects are walking very close each other a big margin of error may arise, that can be reduced with a proper radar calibration. However, the performance of the radar is a compromise between all the configuration parameters and depends on the hardware limits of the system used, and therefore it is not possible to obtain at the same time a high radar visibility range and a high discrimination capacity of nearby objects. At the same time, the garden considered is a very dense environment with various obstacles that interfere with the acquisitions, thus making it difficult to extract information relating to the subjects from the received signal, which in this particular case move slowly. The evaluation of how much time a person has stayed in a specific location can be based on the association of the coordinates for each frame with the frame time.

As described in Sect. 2.2, the GPS data provided by the smartwatches can be processed through the commercial software provided by the vendor and through the custom software developed by the authors, both methods which provide very similar results. In Fig. 8 the paths obtained with two smartwatches of the same model worn by two different people walking very close to each other are represented. It is evident from the figure that the two paths are different in more points. In fact, even if the two smartwatches are very close to each other, the different positions on the arms of the two people, and the attenuation of the Radio Frequency due to trees and buildings on the perimeter, lead to different reception conditions of GPS satellite signals, thus providing different results.

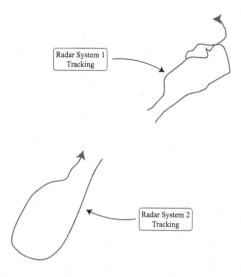

Fig. 7. Example result for the radar system tracking, for only one person in the garden.

A comparison of all the methods described above is depicted in Fig. 9. From the figure is possible to see a good matching of the methods, all providing good performances in tracking the position of the subjects. As introduced above, the main differences are due to the characteristics of the measurements area where

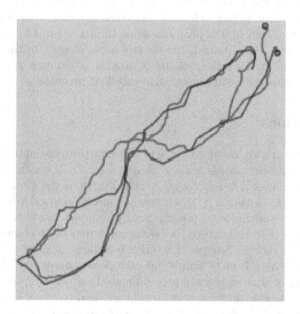

Fig. 8. Result obtained with the GPS for two people walking inside the garden. The blue line is related to the cloud processing and the red line to the custom developed processing. (Color figure online)

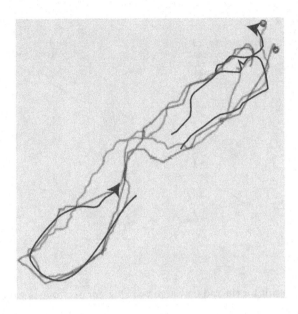

Fig. 9. Comparison between all the methods applied, the green line are the radar systems results, the blue line GPS data processed on cloud and the red with the custom-developed software. (Color figure online)

walls, fences, and trees reduce the radar performances and the GPS performances. However, the tested technological system appears to be appropriate for the purposes envisaged by the project's aims. In fact, even if in the presence of differences in the paths obtained, the sensory areas identify in the garden some macro-sectors within which the presence or absence of patients, and the duration of their presence, can be determined with excellent precision.

5   Conclusions

In this work, a mmWave radar system and two smartwatches equipped with GPS are used to monitoring people inside a garden area. Each system can detect the position and provides information about which area of the garden is preferred by the people who frequent it. Each method provides good performance but the radar system suffers issues coming from the object inside the area such as trees and fences. For this reason, a background removal technique is applied to facilitate the tracking process. The GPS technique is more reliable and the processing of the data is more simple but each person must wear the device and synchronization of all the systems can be difficult. In conclusion, the radar system can detect the targets, the processing technique used to study the environment can be implemented directly on the device and the privacy of each subject can also be preserved. With the smartwatch, the analysis is easier as the information is provided by the GPS but this solution requires each person to wear the device, and that the data is downloaded daily from the smartwatch, which must be frequently recharged anyway.

Acknowledgment. This work is supported by Fondazione Cariverona-Italy in implementation of the financial programme "Bando Programmi riabilitativi 2018", project "AnzianAbili 3.0" (Integrated socio-health rehabilitation paths through technologies for the maintenance and recovery of the residual abilities of vulnerable elderly).

References

1. Amin, M.G., Zhang, Y.D., Ahmad, F., Ho, K.D.: Radar signal processing for elderly fall detection: the future for in-home monitoring. IEEE Sig. Process. Mag. **33**(2), 71–80 (2016)
2. Bouwmans, T., El Baf, F., Vachon, B.: Background modeling using mixture of gaussians for foreground detection-a survey. Recent Patents Comput. Sci. **1**(3), 219–237 (2008)
3. Difrancesco, S., et al.: Out-of-home activity recognition from GPS data in schizophrenic patients. In: 2016 IEEE 29th International Symposium on Computer-Based Medical Systems (CBMS), pp. 324–328. IEEE (2016)
4. Brown, D., Christian, W., Hanson, R.M.: Tracker video analysis and modeling tool (2008). https://physlets.org/tracker/. Accessed 28 July 2021
5. Ester, M., Kriegel, H.P., Sander, J., Xu, X., et al.: A density-based algorithm for discovering clusters in large spatial databases with noise. In: KDD, vol. 96, pp. 226–231 (1996)
6. Texas Instruments: imaging radar using cascaded mmWave sensor reference design (2020)
7. Jankiraman, M.: FMCW Radar Design. Artech House, Boston (2018)
8. Lamard, L., Chapuis, R., Boyer, J.P.: A comparison of two different tracking algorithms is provided for real application. In: 2012 IEEE Intelligent Vehicles Symposium, pp. 414–419. IEEE (2012)
9. Li, G., et al.: Pioneer study on near-range sensing with 4D MIMO-FMCW automotive radars. In: 2019 20th International Radar Symposium (IRS), pp. 1–10. IEEE (2019)
10. Liu, C., Gonzalez, H.A., Vogginger, B., Mayr, C.G.: Phase-based doppler disambiguation in TDM and BPM MIMO FMCW radars. In: 2021 IEEE Radio and Wireless Symposium (RWS), pp. 87–90 (2021). https://doi.org/10.1109/RWS50353.2021.9360348
11. Meinel, H.H.: Evolving automotive radar-from the very beginnings into the future. In: The 8th European Conference on Antennas and Propagation (EuCAP 2014), pp. 3107–3114. IEEE (2014)
12. Patole, S.M., Torlak, M., Wang, D., Ali, M.: Automotive radars: a review of signal processing techniques. IEEE Sig. Process. Mag. **34**(2), 22–35 (2017)
13. Senigagliesi, L., Ciattaglia, G., Gambi, E.: Contactless walking recognition based on mmWave RADAR. In: 2020 IEEE Symposium on Computers and Communications (ISCC), pp. 1–4 (2020). https://doi.org/10.1109/ISCC50000.2020.9219565
14. Shin, D., Shin, D., Shin, D.: Ubiquitous health management system with watch-type monitoring device for dementia patients. J. Appl. Math. **2014** (2014)
15. Sit, Y.L., Li, G., Manchala, S., Afrasiabi, H., Sturm, C., Lubbert, U.: BPSK-based MIMO FMCW automotive-radar concept for 3D position measurement. In: 2018 15th European Radar Conference (EuRAD), pp. 289–292. IEEE (2018)

16. Spinsante, S., Poli, A., Pirani, S., Gioacchini, L.: Lora evaluation in mobility conditions for a connected smart shoe measuring physical activity. In: 2019 IEEE International Symposium on Measurements & Networking (M&N), pp. 1–5. IEEE (2019)
17. Strohm, K., Bloecher, H.L., Schneider, R., Wenger, J.: Development of future short range radar technology. In: European Radar Conference 2005. EURAD 2005, pp. 165–168 (2005). https://doi.org/10.1109/EURAD.2005.1605591
18. Zanaj, E., Disha, D., Spinsante, S., Gambi, E.: A wearable fall detection system based on LoRa LPWAN technology. J. Commun. Softw. Syst. **16**(3), 232–242 (2020)

IoT-Enabled Analysis of Subjective Sound Quality Perception Based on Out-of-Lab Physiological Measurements

Nefeli Dourou, Angelica Poli$^{(\boxtimes)}$ ⓘ, Alessandro Terenzi ⓘ, Stefania Cecchi ⓘ, and Susanna Spinsante ⓘ

Department of Information Engineering, Università Politecnica delle Marche, 60131 Ancona, Italy
{n.a.dourou,a.poli,a.terenzi,s.cecchi,s.spinsante}@staff.univpm.it

Abstract. Sound systems are usually evaluated by means of subjective listening tests that allow to analyze the sound perception from the listener's point of view. In several situations and domains, listening tests can be expensive and complex to arrange, and different variables may influence their reliability, such as ambiguous terminology or contextual biases. To help mitigate these aspects, an analysis of subjective sound quality perception enabled by an Internet of Things - based approach is presented in this paper, exploiting the out-of-lab measurement of physiological parameters by means of a wearable device. In particular, a possible correlation between the subjective assessment of perceived sound quality and the variations of the Inter Beat Interval (IBI) in the cardiac activity of the listeners is analyzed, reporting the measurements performed by a wrist-worn device.

Keywords: Wearable device · Sound stimuli · Physiological signals · Sound quality perception

1 Introduction

Sounds and sound perception play a key role in human life as they allow to communicate with others, by means of speech and music, and also enable self-alerting and orienting when new conditions or events take place [16,27]. The same happens also in the animal kingdom: as an example, sounds are among the most relevant communication strategies for insects and bees [26].

Supported by Marche Region in implementation of the financial programme POR MARCHE FESR 2014–2020, project "Miracle" (Marche Innovation and Research fAcilities for Connected and sustainable Living Environments), CUP B28I19000330007.

S. Spinsante et al. (Eds.): HealthyIoT 2021, LNICST 432, pp. 153–165, 2022.
https://doi.org/10.1007/978-3-030-99197-5_13

In humans, sounds generate reactions, usually in the form of emotions, the classification of which is a powerful tool for a wide range of applications, spanning from industrial to medical ones [14]. In initial studies aimed at investigating the human reactions to acoustic stimuli, the perceived emotions were evaluated by means of self-reports, facial expression and speech analytic [23]. However, these tools were not completely reliable to detect and classify the emotional changes perceived by subjects, and new approaches and analyses were developed, exploiting physiological signals processing. In fact, compared with facial expression, physiological signals represent a more reliable approach to probe the internal cognitive and emotional changes of users, even the hidden ones [5]. For this reason, in the last decades, researchers have tried to develop methods for the automatic recognition of individuals' emotional arousal, starting from the physiological changes [25]. Indeed, since the Autonomic Nervous System (ANS) regulates the emotions producing variations in Heart Rate (HR), respiration rate and sweat secretion, the physiological changes are considered reliable to examine the psychological and emotional statuses of subjects [1].

The collection of physiological signals and the analysis of the variations induced by acoustic stimuli may be applied not only with the aim to recognize the corresponding evoked emotions, but also to develop automatic and quantitative approaches to classify the subjective sound quality perceived by the listeners [19]. Sound quality metrics can be classified into those that quantify some objective aspects of the sound (e.g., pressure level and frequency content) and those that try to quantify the sound effect at the listener's ear (e.g., impression of loudness, tone etc.). In general, subjective testing may involve a single person or many people; it includes the following steps: (i) presentation of sounds to listeners, (ii) judgment of those sounds from the listeners, based on the use of proper standardized scales, and finally (iii) appropriate statistical analysis on the obtained scores. Rigorous perceptual assessment has to be performed according to several standards, including ITU-R BS.1116-1 [9], ITU-R BS.1534-1 [10], and ITU-R BS.1284-2 [11], which define criteria for the selection of the listening panel, describe the test methodology and procedure, and also specify the statistical methods to elaborate the acquired data. Care has to be taken to prevent biased results, for example due to the context, which encompasses both the expectation and emotional state of the listener. In this sense, the acquisition of physiological signals from subjects, before starting the tests, creates the so-called baseline condition, hence the variations induced by the following sound quality perception may be quantified with respect to such a reference status, to limit the impact of bias as much as possible.

Subjective sound quality evaluation performed by means of efficient procedures could be very useful in several application fields, for example all those related to product sound design and quality evaluation (e.g., for appliances or electric vehicles): suitable and effective methods to quantify product sound quality could lead to great advances in the assessment process, and time-consuming studies involving test subjects could be replaced by objective models [4]. An additional advantage would be associated to the possibility of performing such type of tests by using wearable devices to collect physiological signals, instead of desk and laboratory equipment, that may be hard to move and adapt to different testing scenarios. Among the several applications and opportunities of the Internet of Things (IoT)-oriented technologies [13], the IoT devices, especially the wearable ones, support and enable the out-of-lab real-time collection of multimodal physiological data from subjects exposed to sounds and acoustic stimuli, in realistic and unconstrained conditions [24]. Based on the above considerations, this study focuses on the use of a wearable device, the IoT-enabled Empatica E4 multi-sensor wrist-worn one [6], to collect a number of physiological signals, aimed at the investigation of the variations associated to the perceived sound quality, tested from 15 subjects listening to six different types of audio tracks. In particular, the current work extends the preliminary findings presented in [19] and [18], which considered a few subjects, with the aim to explore possible correlations between the perceived sound quality and the variations of the Inter Beat Interval (IBI) in the cardiac activity of the listening subjects, measured by a wrist-worn device. Despite a not-so-huge test population, the outcomes confirm that listening to an audio track always triggers a reaction in the listener. Such response may be detected and recorded through a PPG sensor onboard an IoT-enabled wrist-worn device, allowing the analysis of the average IBI variation, and the corresponding quantitative evaluation of the perceived sound quality.

The paper is organized as follows: Sect. 2 presents the measuring device and the data collection protocol used in the study, while Sect. 3 gives details about the applied data processing procedure. Section 4 presents and discusses the experimental results obtained, and finally, Sect. 5 concludes the paper.

2 Materials and Methods

2.1 Measuring Device

As mentioned above, data collection was performed by using the Empatica E4 multi-sensor wearable device, the most relevant characteristics of which follow:

- Photoplethysmographic (PPG) sensor (sampling frequency: 64 Hz; resolution: 0.9 nW/Digit), measures the Blood Volume Pulse (BVP), from which heart-related parameters, namely the HR, Heart Rate Variability (HRV) and IBI, may be derived;
- 3-axis MEMS Accelerometer (sampling frequency: 32 Hz; resolution: 8 bit of the selected range), measures the continuous gravitational force (g) acting on each of the three spatial directions (X, Y and Z axes);
- Electrodermal Activity (EDA) sensor (sampling frequency: 4 Hz; resolution: 1 digit~900 picoSiemens), measures the skin conductance changes related to Sympathetic Nervous System (SNS) arousal;
- Infrared (IR) Thermopile (sampling frequency: 4 Hz; resolution: 0.02 °C), measures the Skin Temperature (SKT) values.

In this study, data generated from all the available sensors were collected. However, only the HRV signals gathered by the PPG sensors were used for further investigation. The reason is that the HRV is considered the most meaningful indicator of the presence of an acoustic stimulus [3], and more in general, it is one of the most valid indicators of the autonomic regulation for the cardiac function, in response to any external stimuli [17].

2.2 Data Acquisition Protocol

The data collection process applied in each acquisition session is graphically shown in Fig. 1.

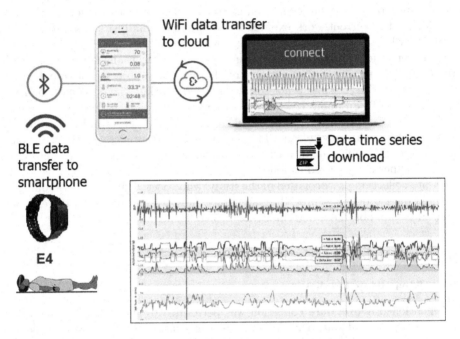

Fig. 1. The E4 IoT-enabled physiological data acquisition process: following the measuring session, data can be downloaded from the Empatica Connect cloud platform.

Experimental tests involved a listener panel of 15 participants (9 males and 6 females, aged between 18 and 60 years), referred to as S1 to S15 in this paper. Each of them performed six test sessions including the following steps:

– *Baseline acquisition* $[t_0; t_1]$: the subject stands in a quiet and relaxed condition for 10 min, during which the physiological parameters are collected. The corresponding signals provide the reference baseline condition;
– *Listening to audio clip* $[t_1; t_2]$: the subject listens to a 40 s-long audio clip, representing the acoustic stimulus in response to which a change in the physiological values is expected;

– *Paper-based evaluation* $[t_2; t_3]$: in the 3 min following the audio clip, the subject is requested to fill in two paper-based evaluation sheets. Firstly, the 100-point continuous quality linear scale (CQS) divided into five-grade sub-scales labelled (from the lowest to the highest) as: bad, poor, fair, good and excellent, as mentioned in the ITU-R norms; secondly, the 9-point Self-Assessment Manikin (SAM) [2] questionnaire to rate the valence and arousal evoked by the external stimulus, by a pictorial tool.

Based on the above description, it follows that each experiment includes a pre-stimulus phase (referred to as *baseline*) lasting 10 min, and a post-stimulus phase (referred to as *reaction to stimulus*), which includes 40 s of audio stimulation, and 3 min without stimulation. Six audio tracks, different in terms of valence (i.e., pleasant and unpleasant), were proposed to each subject: (a) buzzing bees (i.e., buzz of bee swarm), (b) music (i.e., electric guitar and piano cover), (c) distorted music (i.e., distorted electric guitar and piano cover), (d) white noise (i.e., random noise with equal amplitude at different frequencies), (e) rain (i.e., falling rain), and (f) snoring (i.e., human snoring). Each sound was played through headphones to reduce possible subject's distraction during the test.

The time sequence of steps described above is shown in Fig. 2: during all the experiment, the IBI values are measured from the subject, by the Empatica E4.

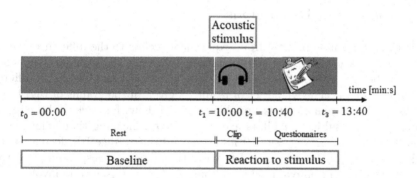

Fig. 2. Time sequence of the IBI measurement steps arranged in the data acquisition protocol.

3   Data Processing

Each element in the IBI parameter values series, for each subject, is obtained as the time distance (in seconds) between two consecutive peaks founded in the corresponding BVP signal, generated by the PPG sensor onboard the E4, which is measured on the wrist and reflects the peripheral blood circulation. Such a process is described in Fig. 3.

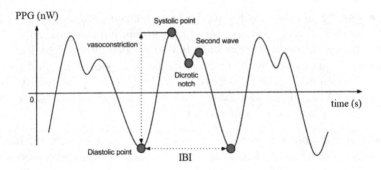

Fig. 3. Computation of IBI values from the signal generated by the PPG sensor (elaborated from https://support.empatica.com/).

For each recording, the average IBI measured during both the *reaction to stimulus* and the *baseline* acquisition (pre-stimulus condition) intervals were computed, and their difference (denoted by *Delta* and measured in seconds) considered to evaluate their corresponding physiological variation due to the specific audio track listening.

4   Results and Discussions

A first set of results obtained from experiments refers to the difference (*Delta*) between the average IBI values measured following the stimulus and those obtained before the stimulus, evaluated for each subject and for the six different audio tracks used. The whole set of results is given in the graphs of Fig. 4.

As a general remark, it is possible to notice how, for each audio clip, the majority of the subjects exhibits a positive *Delta*, meaning that following the acoustic stimulus, the average IBI increases and the average HR decreases. The highest increase of the average IBI (greater than 0.06 s, corresponding to a variation of the HR of approximately 3.6 bpm) is obtained from tests involving the (a) *bees*, (d) *white noise* and (e) *rain* audio tracks, for different subjects (S8, S15 and S14, respectively). Typically, the increase of IBI values, and consequently the decrease of HR ones, indicates effective relaxation state [22]. This trend is mostly evident for those cases in which the frequency of positive *Delta* values over the whole population is high, namely when the participants listen to the (a) *buzzing bees*, (b) *music* and (d) *white noise* tracks. This means that the listeners were in a relatively relaxed state. A preliminary insight shows that, contrarily to what often can be thought, the *buzzing bees* and the *white noise* sounds can have a relaxing effect on the listeners, probably because both the sounds have the same intensity, and constant variance during all the track duration. Being both these sounds evaluated as pleasing, they are often promoted for raising the serenity in the listener. In fact, many researchers recommend the 'contact with

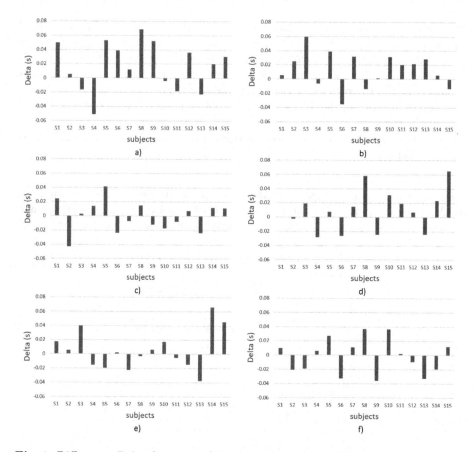

Fig. 4. Difference *Delta* (in seconds) between the average IBI measured after and before the stimulus, for each subject and for the six audio tracks used in experiments with listeners: (a) bees, (b) music, (c) distorted music, (d) white noise, (e) rain, and (f) snoring.

nature' in order to experience the sounds of birds or insects [15,21]; similarly in [8], the authors used the white noise for reducing anxiety in coronary care patients. Concerning the *music* clip, the reason can be referred to the fame of the pop song proposed during the tests.

On the other hand, the decrease of the average IBI value with respect to the baseline is often associated to a stress condition, showing that the subject is stimulated by an external and/or internal event [12]. This is what happens in some cases of our study, where the post-stimulus average IBI decrease is also present, mostly for the (c) *distorted music* (7 subjects out of 15), (e) *rain* (7 subjects out of 15) and (f) *snoring* (7 subjects out of 15) audio clips. These acoustic stimuli determine a reduction of the average IBI, so an increase of the subjects' average HR, even if, again, it does not always happen for the same subject. The maximum decrease of the average IBI is 0.05 s (found only for track (a) in subject S4), corresponding to an average increase of the HR of approximately 3 bpm. As expected, the stress condition is mostly moved by the sound tracks typically perceived as annoying ones. Generally, the sound of rain is associated to a relaxing condition [28], however both the storm and the thunder included in the (e) *rain* track may have modified the general user's emotional perception, activating the SNS and causing an increase of average HR in almost half of the subjects.

The same results may be looked at from the perspective of each subject, as given in Table 1.

Table 1. IBI variation (*Delta*) for each subject involved in tests, and for each audio track: (a) bees, (b) music, (c) distorted music, (d) white noise, (e) rain, and (f) snoring. Symbols: + means positive variation, − negative variation, and 0 no variation.

Track / Subject	(a)	(b)	(c)	(d)	(e)	(f)
S1	+	+	+	0	+	+
S2	+	+	−	+	+	−
S3	−	+	+	+	+	−
S4	−	−	+	−	−	+
S5	+	+	+	+	−	+
S6	+	−	−	−	+	−
S7	+	+	−	+	−	+
S8	+	−	+	+	−	+
S9	+	+	−	−	+	−
S10	−	+	−	+	+	+
S11	−	+	−	+	−	+
S12	+	+	+	+	−	−
S13	−	+	−	−	−	−
S14	+	+	+	+	+	−
S15	+	−	+	+	+	+

From this point of view, it is evident as the S1 is an outlier with no variation between the baseline acquisition and the reaction to the (d) *white noise* stimulus. All the other subjects exhibit either positive or negative variations between the two acquisition time intervals. As an example, subjects S4, S6 and S13 show a prevalent decrease of the average IBI, so they exhibit an increase of their HR for at least 4 out of 6 audio tracks. The track (d) *white noise* is the only one which gives a reduction of the average IBI for all these three subjects.

Moreover, regarding the (a) *buzzing bees*, it can be noticed that all females (S1, S5, S7, S8, S9, S15) presented a positive *Delta*, while for males a few of them (S2, S6, S12, S14). Similarly, the majority of males (S2, S3, S6, S12, S13, S14) presented a decrease of average IBI value listening the *snoring* track, against only one female (S9) out of six.

During experiments, subjects were asked to fill in a paper-based evaluation of the perceived sound quality (CQS evaluation), joint with classification labels generated by using the standardized SAM scale, to identify themselves with five different pictographs (scoring from 1 to 9) over two dimensions, namely Valence and Arousal. The results obtained are shown in Fig. 5, for each audio track and for all the subjects involved in tests. As it is evident, the (c) *distorted music* sound track is mostly evaluated as bad or poor sound quality (dots color is red or orange) by 3 subjects (S4, S13 and S5) who scored an Arousal lower than 5 (corresponding to neutral score), while higher than 5 in 6 subjects. On the other hand, the Valence is perceived differently among the participants: the score is lower than 5 in 6 subjects, higher than 5 in other 6 subjects and equal to 5 in 3 subjects. Oppositely, the (b) *music* exhibits only positive (i.e., good or excellent) evaluation (dots color is blue or green) of the perceived sound quality, while (e) *rain* and (f) *snoring* exhibit mostly positive evaluation (with the exception of two fair evaluations -dots color is grey- given by S3 and S14, respectively). In particular, (b) and (e) show a very high Valence score (especially (b) for which all the subjects gave a score higher than 5, while in (e) two subjects - S2 and S9 - declared both low Valence and Arousal). Concerning the (a) and (d) tracks, the wide spread of dots, in terms of color and position in the plane, represents an obvious different perception of both the quality and evoked emotion by the participants.

Tracks associated to the lowest frequency of positive *Delta* values (see Fig. 4) were evaluated by all the participants as of good/excellent sound quality (i.e., (e) *rain* and (f) *snoring*) or bad/poor sound quality (i.e. (c) *distorted music*). This implies that sounds with a perceived good or bad quality are more likely to be associated to a decrease of average IBI, thus an increase of average HR, than sounds for which quality evaluation is blurred and diverges among the participants. However, the *Music* clip represents an exception. Indeed, although the sound quality was evaluated by all participants as good/excellent, 11 subjects out of 15 (highest frequency) presented positive *Delta* values. As mentioned above, a possible motivation is related to the emotional effects induced by the fame of the pop song proposed.

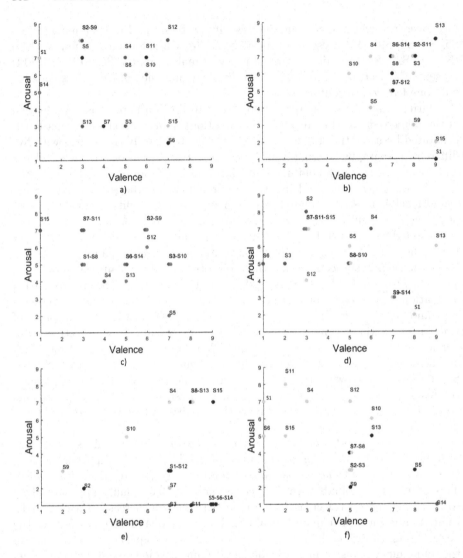

Fig. 5. Valence and Arousal assessment by SAM scale (values from 1 to 9), joint with CQS evaluation (dot color: red = bad (0–20), orange = poor (20–40), grey = fair (40–60), green = good (60–80), blue = excellent (80–100)), for all the subjects and the different audio tracks: (a) bees, (b) music, (c) distorted music, (d) white noise, (e) rain, and (f) snoring. (Color figure online)

5   Conclusion

This paper presented the preliminary results obtained on a population of 15 test listeners involved in the evaluation of the perceived sound quality of six different audio tracks. Such evaluation has been performed by measuring the changes in physiological parameters related to the cardiac activity of each listener, by means of a wearable and IoT-enabled device.

First of all, it is possible to say that listening to an audio track almost always generates a reaction in the listener: the *Delta* between the average IBI values measured following the stimulus, and those obtained before the stimulus, equals zero in just one case out of 90 tests run in total. Then, as a second remark, it is shown how some audio tracks are related to an increase of *Delta*, corresponding to a relaxing effect, and others are associated to a reduction of *Delta*, i.e., a stressing stimulation. It is of interest to observe how different natural sounds, such as buzzing *bees* and *rain*, exhibit opposite reactions from the listeners: relaxing the former, and stressing the latter. Probably, this trend is influenced by the nature of the two sound clips proposed. Indeed, concerning the (a) buzzing *bees* stimulus, this sound can be associated to constant variance in time, like the white noise, that is considered relaxing; on the other hand, during the (e) *rain* stimulus a thunderstorm, an event that generally scares and stresses individuals, arises suddenly.

Secondly, we investigated a possible relationship between the emotional reaction evoked by each audio track, and evaluated by the Valence-Arousal quantification through the SAM scale, and the corresponding CQS scoring, which is typically applied in sound quality tests according to specific technical recommendations. While it is not possible, at this stage, to obtain a general conclusion regarding the different audio tracks, we can observe how sounds with a commonly perceived good or bad quality are more likely to be associated to a decrease of average IBI, than sounds for which quality evaluation diverges, despite being associated to a quite different perception of the evoked emotions by the participants.

The importance of the investigated aspects is clear in the healthcare context. Music is quite often used to ensure the well-being in several daily settings (e.g., home, shops and hospitals), working as therapy or support to reduce stress, anxiety, patient's pain and improve the quality of sleep [7,8,20].

The preliminary results presented in this paper motivate the further development of this research, aimed at increasing the population of listeners participating in test sessions, to reinforce the findings and to achieve more general conclusions about the relationship between perceived sound quality and measurable changes in physiological parameters. Moreover, a multimodal physiological system (including, for example, skin conductance, heart rate variability and temperature) may help in improving the outcomes of the evaluation.

References

1. Bota, P., Wang, C., Fred, A., Silva, H.: Emotion assessment using feature fusion and decision fusion classification based on physiological data: are we there yet? Sensors **20**(17), 4723 (2020)
2. Bradley, M.M., Lang, P.J.: Measuring emotion: the self-assessment manikin and the semantic differential. J. Behav. Ther. Exp. Psychiatry **25**(1), 49–59 (1994)

3. Cosoli, G., Poli, A., Scalise, L., Spinsante, S.: Measurement of multimodal physiological signals for stimulation detection by wearable devices. Measurement **184**, 109966 (2021)
4. Dal Palù, D., De Giorgi, C., Lerma, B., Buiatti, E.: State of the art on the topic. In: Dal Palù, D., De Giorgi, C., Lerma, B., Buiatti, E. (eds.) Frontiers of Sound in Design. SAST, pp. 1–7. Springer, Cham (2018). https://doi.org/10.1007/978-3-319-76870-0_1
5. Dzedzickis, A., Kaklauskas, A., Bucinskas, V.: Human emotion recognition: review of sensors and methods. Sensors **20**(3), 592 (2020)
6. Empatica Inc.: Empatica E4. https://www.empatica.com/en-eu/research/e4/. Accessed Apr 2021
7. Foster, B., Pearson, S., Berends, A., Mackinnon, C.: The expanding scope, inclusivity, and integration of music in healthcare: recent developments, research illustration, and future direction. Healthcare **9**(1) (2021). https://doi.org/10.3390/healthcare9010099. https://www.mdpi.com/2227-9032/9/1/99
8. Hanser, S.B., Mandel, S.E.: The effects of music therapy in cardiac healthcare. Cardiol. Rev. **13**(1), 18–23 (2005)
9. International Telecommunications Union: Methods for the subjective assessment of small impairments in audio system including multichannel sound systems, ITU-R BS.1116-1 (1997)
10. International Telecommunications Union: Method for subjective listening tests of intermediate audio quality, ITU-R Recommendation BS.1534 (2003)
11. International Telecommunications Union: General methods for the subjective assessment of sound quality, ITU-R BS.1284-2 (2019)
12. Jaafar, R., Chung Xian, O.: Analysis of heart rate variability using wearable device. In: Alfred, R., Iida, H., Haviluddin, H., Anthony, P. (eds.) Computational Science and Technology. LNEE, vol. 724, pp. 453–461. Springer, Singapore (2021). https://doi.org/10.1007/978-981-33-4069-5_37
13. John Dian, F., Vahidnia, R., Rahmati, A.: Wearables and the Internet of Things (IoT), applications, opportunities, and challenges: a survey. IEEE Access **8**, 69200–69211 (2020)
14. Kołodziej, M., Tarnowski, P., Majkowski, A., Rak, R.: Electrodermal activity measurements for detection of emotional arousal. Bull. Pol. Acad. Sci. Tech. Sci. **67**(4), 813–826 (2019)
15. Maller, C., Townsend, M., Pryor, A., Brown, P., St Leger, L.: Healthy nature healthy people: 'contact with nature' as an upstream health promotion intervention for populations. Health Promot. Int. **21**(1), 45–54 (2005). https://doi.org/10.1093/heapro/dai032
16. Oxenham, A.J.: How we hear: the perception and neural coding of sound. Ann. Rev. Psychol. **69**(1), 27–50 (2018). pMID: 29035691
17. Parizek, D., Sladicekova, K., Tonhajzerova, I., Veterník, M., Jakus, J.: The effect of music on heart rate variability. Acta Medica Martiniana **21**(1), 1–8 (2021)
18. Poli, A., Brocanelli, A., Cecchi, S., Orcioni, S., Spinsante, S.: Preliminary results of IoT-enabled EDA-based analysis of physiological response to acoustic stimuli. In: Goleva, R., Garcia, N.R.C., Pires, I.M. (eds.) HealthyIoT 2020. LNICST, vol. 360, pp. 124–136. Springer, Cham (2021). https://doi.org/10.1007/978-3-030-69963-5_9
19. Poli, A., Cecchi, S., Spinsante, S., Terenzi, A., Bettarelli, F.: A preliminary study on the correlation between subjective sound quality perception and physiological parameters. In: Audio Engineering Society Convention 150, May 2021

20. Rahman, J.S., Gedeon, T., Caldwell, S., Jones, R., Jin, Z.: Towards effective music therapy for mental health care using machine learning tools: human affective reasoning and music genres. J. Artif. Intell. Soft Comput. Res. **11**(1), 5–20 (2021)
21. Ratcliffe, E.: Sound and soundscape in restorative natural environments: a narrative literature review. Front. Psychol. **12**, 963 (2021)
22. The, A.-F., Reijmerink, I., van der Laan, M., Cnossen, F.: Heart rate variability as a measure of mental stress in surgery: a systematic review. Int. Arch. Occup. Environ. Health **93**(7), 805–821 (2020). https://doi.org/10.1007/s00420-020-01525-6
23. Samadiani, N., et al.: A review on automatic facial expression recognition systems assisted by multimodal sensor data. Sensors **19**(8), 1863 (2019)
24. Segura-Garcia, J., Calero, J.M.A., Pastor-Aparicio, A., Marco-Alaez, R., Felici-Castell, S., Wang, Q.: 5G IoT system for real-time psycho-acoustic soundscape monitoring in smart cities with dynamic computational offloading to the edge. IEEE Internet Things J. **8**(15), 12467–12475 (2021)
25. Suzuki, K., Laohakangvalvit, T., Matsubara, R., Sugaya, M.: Constructing an emotion estimation model based on EEG/HRV indexes using feature extraction and feature selection algorithms. Sensors **21**(9), 2910 (2021)
26. Terenzi, A., Cecchi, S., Spinsante, S.: On the importance of the sound emitted by honey bee hives. Vet. Sci. **7**(4), 168 (2020)
27. Terenzi, A., Spinsante, S., Cecchi, S.: Review on electric vehicles exterior noise generation and evaluation. In: 2020 AEIT International Conference of Electrical and Electronic Technologies for Automotive (AEIT Automotive 2020), pp. 1–6 (2020). https://doi.org/10.23919/AEITAUTOMOTIVE50086.2020.9307397
28. Yu, B., Hu, J., Funk, M., Feijs, L.: A study on user acceptance of different auditory content for relaxation, October 2016. https://doi.org/10.1145/2986416.2986418

CS-Based Decomposition of Acoustic Stimuli-Driven GSR Peaks Sensed by an IoT-Enabled Wearable Device

Federico Casaccia, Grazia Iadarola$^{(\boxtimes)}$ ⓘ, Angelica Poli$^{(\boxtimes)}$ ⓘ, and Susanna Spinsante ⓘ

Department of Information Engineering, Università Politecnica delle Marche, Ancona 60131, Italy
s1091918@studenti.univpm.it,
{g.iadarola,a.poli,s.spinsante}@staff.univpm.it

Abstract. The Galvanic Skin Response (GSR) signal, measured as the electrical conductance between a pair of electrodes placed over a person's skin, consists of a tonic component superposed by a phasic component. In the GSR phasic component several peaks appear corresponding to specific events. Therefore, the information content of peaks is very useful in a wide range of applications. This work investigates the effectiveness of a decomposition-based Compressed Sensing (CS) approach for extraction of peaks from GSR signals acquired with an IoT-enabled wrist-worn device, during unpleasant sound stimulation. Then, once the sparse peaks are detected, the overall GSR phasic component is reconstructed, too.

Keywords: Galvanic Skin Response · Compressed sensing · IoT-Wearable device · Acoustic stimuli

1 Introduction

Galvanic Skin Response (GSR), also known as ElectroDermal Activity (EDA) or Skin Conductance (SC), is the electrical signal of the sympathetic activity of sweat glands. In detail, GSR is typically recorded as the electric conductance between a pair of electrodes placed over a person's skin, near high density regions of sweat glands (e.g., hand palm or fingertips). The GSR signal is characterized by two main components: (i) a slowly varying tonic component, or SC level (SCL); (ii) a phasic component or SC response (SCR) where several peaks appear corresponding to specific events. The hypothesized connection between variations in a subject's skin conductance and psychological state has been confirmed at the beginning of the 21st century by means of a simultaneous analysis of brain function, using functional Magnetic Resonance Imaging and GSR [10]. In the last decade, wearable devices have given us the opportunity of a non-invasive measure of the GSR signal through simple settings [8].

© ICST Institute for Computer Sciences, Social Informatics and Telecommunications Engineering 2022
Published by Springer Nature Switzerland AG 2022. All Rights Reserved
S. Spinsante et al. (Eds.): HealthyIoT 2021, LNICST 432, pp. 166–179, 2022.
https://doi.org/10.1007/978-3-030-99197-5_14

GSR peaks are difficult to extract from an observed GSR signal for a number of reasons, such as potentially overlapping SCR, or a predominant SCL [29]. In recent years, various signal decomposition approaches have been proposed to overcome these difficulties [1,5,6] but the problem still remains. The conventional approach to evaluate GSR peaks is based on the trough-to-peak detection [25] and it has already been explored depending on three different types of acoustic stimuli in [23]. This work investigates, instead, a Compressed Sensing (CS) [16] approach that exploits the intrinsic sparse nature of peaks. CS is, indeed, a technique able to exploit the signal sparsity in some domains [11–15,22]. As shown in [24], CS exhibits better performance in terms of peak count, if compared to Ledalab automatic toolbox for GSR processing. It is important to consider that not only CS allows to perform a correct count of the number of GSR peaks, but it also works on compressed samples, while automatic toolboxes (such as Ledalab or EDA Explorer) do not implement any compression mechanism. Moreover, compression mechanisms are generally a valid instrument to solve the problems in Internet-of-Things (IoT) paradigm adopted for healthcare monitoring and management (such as big data quantity, security, privacy) [18].

The aim of this work is to investigate the effectiveness of a decomposition-based CS method [26] for reconstruction of GSR phasic component. The method proposed in [26] is firstly evaluated by using synthetically generated signals. Then, the method is analyzed also on GSR signals experimentally acquired by an IoT-enabled wrist-worn device, the Empatica E4 wristband [20], in reaction to unpleasant acoustic stimuli.

The paper is organized as follows: Sect. 2 shortly describes the GSR signal, reviewing the state-of-the-art about GSR signal analysis in time domain with the related issues. Section 3 presents the acquisition IoT-enabled sensing device, the protocol to collect data, as well as the methods used to process it. Section 5 presents and discusses the results obtained. Finally, Sect. 6 concludes the paper.

2   Background

2.1   GSR Signal

The GSR signal is a physiological signal reflecting changes in the electrical properties of the human skin, resulting from the activity of the Sympathetic Nervous System (SNS, a branch of the autonomic nervous system) [17]. As such, GSR values provide an optimal marker of both psychological and physiological arousal, being associated to emotional and cognitive human activities [9].

Research studies have proposed two different approaches to measure GSR signals: the exosomatic method (applying a direct current (DC) or an alternating current (AC)) and the endosomatic method (without applying any external current or voltage) [30]. The former approach is the most commonly used, with an external constant voltage source that is connected to the human skin through electrodes. Generally, a GSR sensing device consists of the following components: two electrodes to collect signal, an amplifier to increase the signal amplitude, and a digitizer to convert analog raw signals into digital form; in the case of a wireless device, also data transmission modules (e.g., Bluetooth or WiFi transceivers) are added for communicating with a recording system [25]. Both the measuring methods mentioned above produce a GSR signal, that can be always decomposed in the two components: SCL and SCR. A single SCR, as shown in Fig. 1 from [3], is characterized by: i) peak amplitude (amplitude difference between the onset and the maximum of the peak - *SCR amplitude*); ii) latency (time interval between the stimulus onset and the GSR peak onset - *SCR latency*); iii) rise time (time interval between the onset and the maximum of the peak - *rise time*); iv) recovery time (time interval from peak to total recovery - *rec.t/2* and *rec.tc*, 50% and 63% recovery respectively).

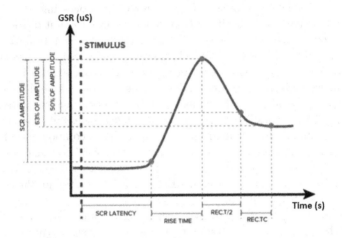

Fig. 1. Shape of a SCR and the related descriptive metrics [3].

2.2   GSR Signal Analysis in Time Domain

For the purpose of both emotion detection and recognition, the GSR signal is one of the most investigated physiological signals. In particular, the response to specific external stimuli, such as audio [23] and video [31], is analysed in time domain in terms of SCR peaks and number of peaks over time.

Among the algorithms developed to analyse the SCR signal, the detection of both SCR peaks and troughs is the most used. Such algorithm identifies a peak or trough, by determining the time-series points where the derivative of the signal is zero; then, the corresponding SCR peaks amplitude and rise-time are computed with respect to the peak onset [1]. However, a weakness of this implementation is evident when short inter-stimulus intervals are established. In fact, it may happen that two close SCR peaks overlap, with the tail of the preceding SCR peak hiding the initial onset of the next SCR peak [21]. A misdetection can result in a distorted estimation of the event-related values, and a pair of events may be detected as a single one. To face this problem, several studies have proposed mathematical models to decompose the GSR signal into its two components. As an example, Alexander et al. [1] proposed an automated analysis based on the mathematical process of deconvolution to extract the phasic activity from the

GSR signal [6]. This approach relies on the physiological assumption, according to which the GSR signal results from a convolution between the sudomotor nerve activity (corresponding to a driver function) exhibiting peaks in response to a stimulus, and an Impulse Response Function (IRF). By deconvolving the GSR signal with a specific IRF, the driver function (sequence of discrete peaks) is revealed, and the peaks can be identified to reconstruct the corresponding SCR [5]. In particular, the IRF depicts the SCR shape resulting from an impulse. In 1987, Schneider et al. [28] modeled the SCR shape with a bi-exponential function, called Bateman function, in which time constants represent the steep onset and slow recovery. However, the inter- and intra- individual variability, that are significantly evident in SCR shape, can affect the performance of this approach [27].

Another GSR signal decomposition method, presented by Benedek and Kaernbach in [6], is based on nonnegative deconvolution, called Discrete Decomposition Analysis (DDA). This approach lies on the nonnegativity of the driver function and maximal compactness of its impulses (i.e. peaks). Same authors also proposed the Continuous Decomposition Analysis (CDA) based on a standard deconvolution algorithm. Both the overmentioned decomposition methods are widely used and freely available in the Ledalab toolbox [4]. In this case, the concept of single and discrete response is replaced by a continuous measure of SCR (i.e. phasic activity - an indicator of sympathetic activity) and a response window (indicator of event-related activity).

3   Materials and Methods

3.1   The IoT-Enabled Sensing Device

Experimental sessions were performed using a single wearable, the Empatica E4 [19], an IoT-enabled and multi-sensor wristband device designed to comfortably acquire in real-time data during everyday life. As specified by the manufacturer, the device hosts four sensors, namely a photoplethysmographic sensor (PPG) sampled at 64 Hz, a 3-axial MEMS accelerometer (sampling frequency, $f_s = 32$ Hz), a GSR sensor ($f_s = 4$ Hz), and an optical thermopile ($f_s = 4$ Hz).

This study only considers the signals generated by the GSR sensor (see Table 1 for further technical details), which measures the electrical conductance of the skin from the bottom of the wrist, by applying an extremely small amount of alternating current between two silver-coated electrodes embedded into the device bracelet.

Experimental tests involving the IoT-enabled E4 device can be conducted in two different modalities: streaming and recording mode, with a claimed battery life >20 hours and >36 hours, respectively. In our study, participants used the Empatica device in real-time streaming mode, connected via Bluetooth Low Energy (BLE) to the mobile App (i.e., E4 realtime) running on a smartphone. The recorded samples are automatically uploaded and safely stored in the E4 Connect cloud-based repository, where also the session duration, device serial

Table 1. Technical specification of the GSR sensor.

Parameter	Value [Units]
Sampling frequency	4 [Hz]
Resolution	1 digit ~900 [pS]
Range	0.01–100 [μS]
Alternating current (max 100 μA) frequency	8 [Hz]

number and session date are available as well. Following the data collection session, data acquired can be downloaded as a compressed folder (.zip), containing one .csv file for each sensor and an additional file (named tags.csv) related to events marked during a session. The overall GSR sensing and data acquisition process is graphically shown in Fig. 2.

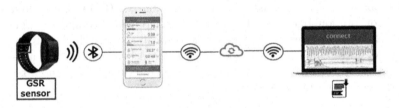

Fig. 2. The E4 IoT-enabled GSR data acquisition process: following the measuring session, data can be retrieved from the Empatica cloud platform.

Concerning the GSR files, data samples given in microSiemens (μS) are listed in a single-column format, after indicating the starting time (t_0, expressed in UTC) of the acquisition process in the first row, and the sampling rate in the second one.

3.2   Data Collection

Six healthy subjects (3 males and 3 females, aged between 20 and 60 years old) were enrolled in this study. Before starting the data collection, participants were briefed on the study procedure, and an informed consent was signed.

To avoid as much as possible any distraction during the signal acquisition sessions, the participants were left alone in their room, and asked to lay on a bed and relax with closed eyes. The E4 was placed on the dominant wrist to acquire the skin electrical signal. Prior to signals registration performed, volunteers were asked to push the event-marker button located on the wristband, at the start and at the end of each acoustic stimulus, to enable the automatic real-time annotation of sessions (in the tags.csv file).

The overall data acquisition lasted about 12 min (see Fig. 3): i) 5 min at resting condition where the physiological reference baseline was collected with the subject relaxed; ii) 2 min (from 05:30 to 07:00 min:s; minutes:seconds) where physiological changes were measured. In particular, sound stimuli were played at 05:30 min:s, 06:30 min:s, and 07:00 min:s through headphones to the subject; iii) 5 min again at resting condition.

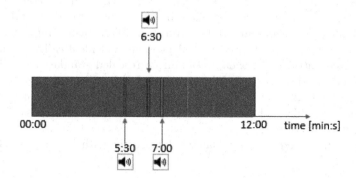

Fig. 3. Schematic representation of the temporal structure of the auditory stimulation sessions presented to the participants.

Audio clips, lasting 6 seconds per each, were extracted from the International Affective Digitized Sounds (IADS-2) database [33], that contains a collection of sounds rated in terms of valence (pleasantness), arousal (intensity of sensations) and dominance (control over sensations) according to the 9-point Self-Assessment Manikin (SAM) scale [7]. Based on the unpleasant valence score, the sounds listed in Table 2 were selected for the current study.

Table 2. Valence, arousal and dominance scores (dimensionless values, mean value $\pm$ standard deviation) of the selected sounds.

Sound (no. IADS)	Valence	Arousal	Dominance
Scream (no. 275)	2.05 ± 1.62	8.16 ± 2.15	2.55 ± 2.01
Car wreck (no. 424)	2.04 ± 1.52	7.99 ± 1.66	2.29 ± 1.74
Buzzer (no. 712)	2.42 ± 1.62	7.98 ± 1.99	2.84 ± 2.11

4   Data Processing

The GSR signal acquired has to be first pre-processed in order to remove noise and possible motion artefacts. Electrical noise is reduced by applying a low-pass filter with a small cut-off frequency (generally <1 Hz), and similarly the motion artefacts with both a low pass filtering and manual inspection of the signal [32]. Once the GSR signal has been pre-processed, it can be decomposed in SCL and SCR components.

4.1   Synthethic GSR Signals

Based on the work by Jain et al. [26], and in order to evaluate the recovery accuracy of the proposed approach, the following parameters were defined:

- impulse response vector $\mathbf{h}$;
- time steps γ and δ;
- approximately sparse vectors $\mathbf{x} \in \mathbf{X}_\delta^s$ and $\mathbf{b} \in \mathbf{B}_\gamma^c$ with a certain number s of peaks and a number c of baseline jumps; $\mathbf{x}$ was obtained by taking the s significant components uniformly at random, filling such components with a random vector (characterized by independent and identically exponentially distributed entries) and then, by adding a rescaled standard Gaussian random vector with l_1 norm δ; $\mathbf{Db}$ was computed by selecting the c significant components uniformly at random, filling such components with a standard Gaussian variable, and then by adding a rescaled standard Gaussian random vector with l_1 norm γ;
- the noise $\mathbf{n}$, as rescaled Gaussian random vector with l_2 norm equal to $\varepsilon = 0.01$;

All these parameters allow to define:

$$\mathbf{Dy} = \mathbf{DT_h x} + \alpha \mathbf{Db} + \mathbf{n}, \tag{1}$$

where α is the scaling factor applied to $\mathbf{Db}$ related to $\mathbf{DT_h x}$ and $\mathbf{T}$ a Toeplitz matrix constructed from the vector $\mathbf{h}$.

5   Test Implementation and Results

To verify the feasibility and accuracy of the proposed CS-based approach, the experimental tests were preliminarily carried out on synthetic GSR signals, for which the amount of SCR peaks was defined *a priori*, and then on real GSR signals to acoustic stimuli of Table 2.

5.1   Preliminary Analysis on Synthetic GSR Signals

In a preliminary analysis the feasibility of CS framework for GSR signals was evaluated on synthetic GSR signals. In this test only the peak vector $\mathbf{x}$ was reconstructed. The figure of merit used to analyze the reconstruction performance is the Recovery Error (RE) [2], defined as the norm of the difference between the original peak vector $\mathbf{x}$ and the reconstructed peak vector $\hat{\mathbf{x}}$, divided by the norm of the original peak vector. Thus, RE can be written as:

$$RE = \frac{\|\mathbf{x} - \hat{\mathbf{x}}\|_2}{\|\mathbf{x}\|_2}. \tag{2}$$

Figure 4 illustrates the RE diagrams obtained for three different values of the scaling factor $\alpha = \{0.01, 0.1, 1\}$. The diagrams were computed depending on the number of SCR peaks chosen in the set $s = \{10, 20, \ldots, 240\}$ and the number of baseline jumps in the set $c = \{10, 20, \ldots, 350\}$. Specifically, 5 synthetic GSR signals were randomly generated for each value of peaks amount in the set s. RE was firstly computed for each synthetic GSR signal and, then, the obtained RE values were averaged. All the possible combinations between peaks and baseline jumps of average RE are reported as colored pixels. The three diagrams show that when scaling the magnitude of the baseline component, through a lower factor α, a lower average RE is obtained.

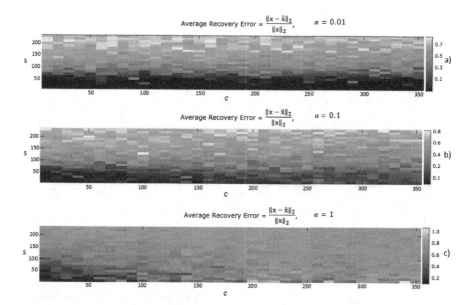

Fig. 4. Diagrams of RE depending on the number of GSR peaks s and baseline jumps c, for three values of the scaling factor α: a) 0.01, b) 0.1, c) 1.

5.2   Test on Real GSR Signals

In the second test the entire phasic component of real GSR signals was recovered. In particular, the phasic component was estimated as the convolution between the reconstructed peak vector $\hat{x}$ and the impulse response vector $\mathbf{h}$, obtained by sampling at 4 *Samples/s* the bi-exponential function:

$$f(u) = 2(e^{-u/\tau_1} - e^{-u/\tau_2})$$ (3)

with $u \in [0, 40]$, $\tau_1 = 10$ and $\tau_2 = 1$.

Figures 5, 6, 7, 8, 9 and 10 show the reconstruction of the phasic component of the GSR signals acquired by 6 subjects, as described in Subsect. 3.2. The figures report all the intermediate signals step-by-step, till the final reconstruction phase. The colored vertical lines indicate the moments when the acoustic stimuli

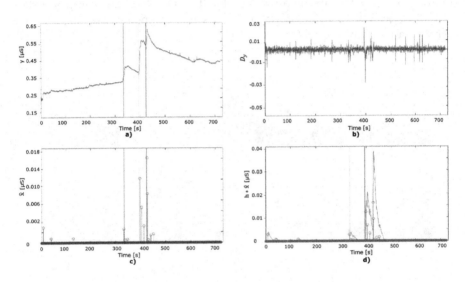

Fig. 5. Step-by-step reconstruction for subject 1.

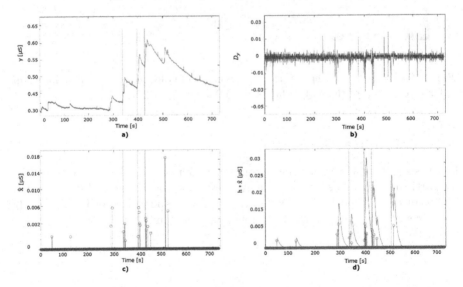

Fig. 6. Step-by-step reconstruction for subject 2.

occurred. In particular, each figure illustrates: a) the acquired GSR signal $\mathbf{y}$; b) the GSR signal filtered by the matrix $\mathbf{D}$; c) the reconstructed peak vector $\hat{\mathbf{x}}$; d) the reconstructed phasic component $\hat{\mathbf{x}} * \mathbf{h}$. The obtained results exhibit a good reconstruction of GSR phasic component for all the 6 subjects.

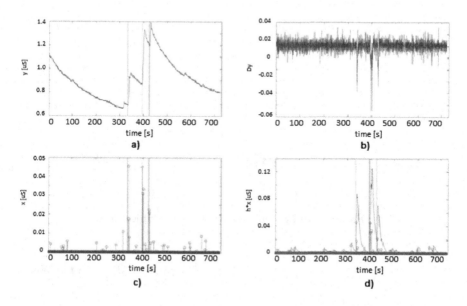

Fig. 7. Step-by-step reconstruction for subject 3.

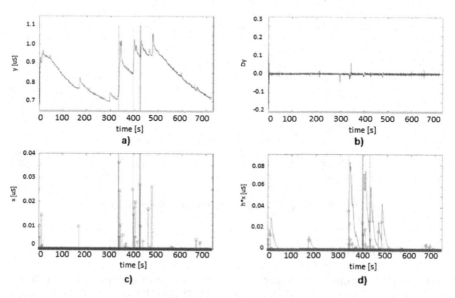

Fig. 8. Step-by-step reconstruction for subject 4.

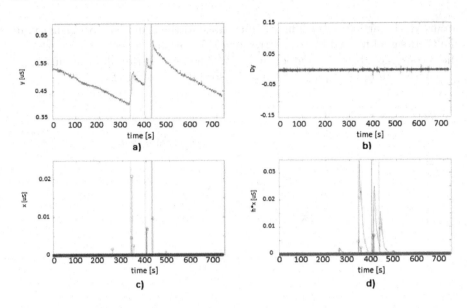

Fig. 9. Step-by-step reconstruction for subject 5.

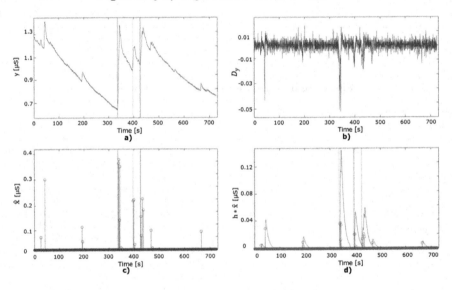

Fig. 10. Step-by-step reconstruction for subject 6.

6   Conclusion

In this work, a decomposition method based on the approach proposed by Jain et al. [26] has been employed, to reconstruct GSR signals through CS framework. In particular, the reconstruction was preliminarly evaluated on peaks of GSR signals that were synthetically generated, in order to verify the feasibility of the decomposition method and its reliability in peaks reconstruction. Subsequently, the reconstruction was tested on real signals, experimentally acquired with a wearable device from 6 subjects, in response to unpleasant acoustic stimuli. In this case, the entire phasic component of the GSR signal was reconstructed. From the obtained results, a good reconstruction of GSR phasic component can be observed. The proposed method could be exploited to analyse the reaction of subjects exposed to unpleasant sounds in the long-term, as it may be the case for workers in constructions or harsh industrial environments.

Future investigations will be devoted to recover the whole GSR signal, including the tonic component, that is determined by several individual factors (e.g. gender and age), irrespective of any stimulus. Besides, future studies will be performed on a bigger set of signals, by involving more subjects as well as other devices for GSR acquisition.

Acknowledgment. The paper was supported by the POR MARCHE FESR 2014-2020 project: *"Marche Innovation and Research fAcilities for Connected and sustainable Living Environments (MIRACLE)"*- CUP B28I19000330007 and by the More Years Better Lives JPI and the Italian Ministero dell'Istruzione, Università e Ricerca within the project *"Privacy-Aware and Acceptable Lifelogging services for older and frail people (PAAL)"* - Grant no: PAAL JTC2017, CUP: I36G17000380001.

References

1. Alexander, D., Trengove, C., Johnston, P., Cooper, T., August, J., Gordon, E.: Separating individual skin conductance responses in a short inter stimulus-interval paradigm. J. Neurosci. Methods **146**(1), 116–123 (2005). https://doi.org/10.1016/j.jneumeth.2005.02.001
2. Arie, R., Brand, A., Engelberg, S.: Compressive sensing and sub-Nyquist sampling. IEEE Instrum. Meas. Mag. **23**(2), 94–101 (2020). https://doi.org/10.1109/MIM.2020.9062696
3. Babaei, E., Tag, B., Dingler, T., Velloso, E.: A critique of electrodermal activity practices at chi. In: Proceedings of the 2021 CHI Conference on Human Factors in Computing Systems. CHI 2021. Association for Computing Machinery, New York (2021). https://doi.org/10.1145/3411764.3445370
4. Benedek, M., Kaernbach, C.: LEDALAB: Open source Matlab software for analysis of skin conductance data (viz. EDA; GSR), September 2010. http://www.ledalab.de/
5. Benedek, M., Kaernbach, C.: A continuous measure of phasic electrodermal activity. J. Neurosci. Methods **190**(1), 80–91 (2010). https://doi.org/10.1016/j.jneumeth.2010.04.028
6. Benedek, M., Kaernbach, C.: Decomposition of skin conductance data by means of nonnegative deconvolution. Psychophysiology **47**(4), 647–658 (2010). https://doi.org/10.1111/j.1469-8986.2009.00972.x
7. Bradley, M.M., Lang, P.J.: Measuring emotion: the self-assessment manikin and the semantic differential. J. Behav. Ther. Exp. Psychiatry **25**(1), 49–59 (1994)
8. Cosoli, G., Iadarola, G., Poli, A., Spinsante, S.: Learning classifiers for analysis of blood volume pulse signals in IoT-enabled systems. In: 2021 IEEE International Workshop on Metrology for Industry 4.0 IoT (MetroInd4.0 IoT), pp. 307–312 (2021)

9. Cowley, B.U., Torniainen, J.: A short review and primer on electrodermal activity in human computer interaction applications (2016)
10. Critchley, H.D., Elliott, R., Mathias, C.J., Dolan, R.J.: Neural activity relating to generation and representation of galvanic skin conductance responses: a functional magnetic resonance imaging study. J. Neurosci. **20**(8), 3033–3040 (2000). https://doi.org/10.1523/JNEUROSCI.20-08-03033.2000
11. Daponte, P., De Vito, L., Iadarola, G., Picariello, F.: ECG monitoring based on dynamic compressed sensing of multi-lead signals. Sensors **21**(21), 7003 (2021)
12. Daponte, P., De Vito, L., Iadarola, G., Picariello, F., Rapuano, S.: Deterministic compressed sensing of heart sound signals. In: 2021 IEEE International Symposium on Medical Measurements and Applications (MeMeA), pp. 1–6 (2021)
13. Daponte, P., De Vito, L., Iadarola, G., Rapuano, S.: PRBS non-idealities affecting random demodulation analog-to-information converters. In: 21st IMEKO TC-4 International Symposium on Understanding the World through Electrical and Electronic Measurement and 19th IMEKO International Workshop on ADC Modelling and Testing, pp. 71–76, September 2016
14. Daponte, P., De Vito, L., Iadarola, G., Rapuano, S.: A reduced-code method for integral nonlinearity testing in DACs. Measurement **182**, 109764 (2021)
15. Daponte, P., Vito, L.D., Iadarola, G., Rapuano, S.: Analog multiplication in random demodulation analog–to–information converters. J. Phys. Conf. Ser. **1065**(5), 052048 (2018)
16. Donoho, D.L.: Compressed sensing. IEEE Trans. Inf. Theor. **52**, 1289–1306 (2006)
17. Dutta, S., Dash, S., Padhy, N.: Analysis of human emotion-based data using MIoT technique. Med. Internet Things Tech. Pract. Appl. 199 (2021)
18. Elhoseny, M., et al.: Security and privacy issues in medical internet of things: overview, countermeasures, challenges and future directions. Sustainability **13**(21), 11645 (2021)
19. Empatica Inc., MI, IT: E4 WristBand from Empatica User's Manual (2018)
20. Garbarino, M., Lai, M., Bender, D., Picard, R.W., Tognetti, S.: Empatica E3 - A wearable wireless multi-sensor device for real-time computerized biofeedback and data acquisition. In: 2014 4th International Conference on Wireless Mobile Communication and Healthcare - Transforming Healthcare Through Innovations in Mobile and Wireless Technologies (MOBIHEALTH), pp. 39–42 (2014). https://doi.org/10.1109/MOBIHEALTH.2014.7015904
21. Grings, W.W., Lockhart, R.A.: Problems of magnitude measurement with multiple GSRs. Psychol. Rep. **17**(3), 979–982 (1965)
22. Iadarola, G.: Characterization of analog-to-information converters. IEEE Instrum. Meas. Mag. **25**(1), 98–99 (2022)
23. Iadarola, G., Poli, A., Spinsante, S.: Analysis of galvanic skin response to acoustic stimuli by wearable devices. In: 2021 IEEE International Symposium on Medical Measurements and Applications (MeMeA), pp. 1–6 (2021)
24. Iadarola, G., Poli, A., Spinsante, S.: Reconstruction of galvanic skin response peaks via sparse representation. In: 2021 IEEE International Instrumentation and Measurement Technology Conference (I2MTC), pp. 1–6 (2021)
25. iMotions: EDA/GSR Pocket Guide - iMotions, September 2021. https://imotions.com/guides/eda-gsr/
26. Jain, S., Oswal, U., Xu, K.S., Eriksson, B., Haupt, J.: A compressed sensing based decomposition of electrodermal activity signals. IEEE Trans. Biomed. Eng. **64**(9), 2142–2151 (2017). https://doi.org/10.1109/TBME.2016.2632523
27. Posada-Quintero, H.F., Chon, K.H.: Innovations in electrodermal activity data collection and signal processing: a systematic review. Sensors **20**(2), 479 (2020)

28. Schneider, R.: A mathematical-model of human-skin conductance. Psychophysiology **24**(5), 610 (1987)
29. Silveira, F., Eriksson, B., Sheth, A., Sheppard, A.: Predicting audience responses to movie content from electro-dermal activity signals. In: Proceedings of the 2013 ACM International Joint Conference on Pervasive and Ubiquitous Computing, pp. 707–716. UbiComp 2013. Association for Computing Machinery, New York (2013). https://doi.org/10.1145/2493432.2493508
30. Society for Psychophysiological Research Ad Hoc Committee on Electrodermal Measures: Publication recommendations for electrodermal measurements. Psychophysiology **49**(8), 1017–1034 (2012). https://doi.org/10.1111/j.1469-8986.2012.01384.x
31. Terkildsen, T., Makransky, G.: Measuring presence in video games: an investigation of the potential use of physiological measures as indicators of presence. Int. J. Hum. Comput. Stud. **126**, 64–80 (2019)
32. Topoglu, Y., Watson, J., Suri, R., Ayaz, H.: Electrodermal activity in ambulatory settings: a narrative review of literature. In: Ayaz, H. (ed.) AHFE 2019. AISC, vol. 953, pp. 91–102. Springer, Cham (2020). https://doi.org/10.1007/978-3-030-20473-0_10
33. Yang, W., et al.: Affective auditory stimulus database: an expanded version of the international affective digitized sounds (IADS-E). Behav. Res. Methods **50**, 1415–1429 (2018)

GAIToe: Gait Analysis Utilizing an IMU for Toe Walking Detection and Intervention

Ghazal Ershadi[1], Migyeong Gwak[1(✉)], Jane Liu[1], Gichan Lee[1], Afshin Aminian[2], and Majid Sarrafzadeh[1]

[1] University of California, Los Angeles, Los Angeles, CA 90095, USA
{ghazaalershadi,mgwak,majid}@cs.ucla.edu
[2] Children's Hospital of Orange County, 1201 West La Veta Avenue, Orange, CA 92868, USA

Abstract. Idiopathic toe walking (ITW) is a walking pattern in which a person habitually walks on their forefoot with the absence of heel contact during the gait cycle. Gait rehabilitation can be achieved through behavior modification by employing a wearable device and giving the user immediate feedback. In this paper, we introduce GAIToe, a real-time toe walking detection and intervention platform that remotely monitors walking patterns. GAIToe utilizes an Inertial Measurement Unit (IMU) located in the insole and incorporates a machine learning model to detect different walking, sitting, and standing behaviors. GAIToe identifies these activities with 88% accuracy and provides vibration feedback following consecutive toe strikes. It also provides an Android application to transmit the data and a visual context to monitor the walking patterns. For the preliminary evaluation of GAIToe, we collected activity samples from ten healthy subjects.

Keywords: Idiopathic toe walking · Gait analysis · Wearable sensor · Inertial Measurement Unit (IMU) · Machine learning

1 Introduction

Toe walking is a gait pattern where a person walks on the toes or balls of the feet without the heel touching the ground during the gait cycle. General conditions associated with toe walking include autistic spectrum disorders, cerebral palsy, congenital talipes equinus, developmental coordination disorder, and muscle dystrophy [1, 2]. When children first begin to walk, the presence of toe walking is not unusual; however, the heel-toe gait pattern can become persistent as they grow up [3]. If older children persist in toe walking with no signs of neurological, orthopedic, or psychiatric disease, or the cause of toe walking remains unexplained, they are diagnosed with idiopathic toe walking (ITW) [4,5]. A child with ITW habitually walks on the forefoot, but they can perform heel-toe walk for short periods when they are asked to do so [1,4]. The incidence of ITW has been

© ICST Institute for Computer Sciences, Social Informatics and Telecommunications Engineering 2022
Published by Springer Nature Switzerland AG 2022. All Rights Reserved
S. Spinsante et al. (Eds.): HealthyIoT 2021, LNICST 432, pp. 180–195, 2022.
https://doi.org/10.1007/978-3-030-99197-5_15

estimated at 7% to 24% of the childhood population [6]. Persistent toe walking may induce foot deformities, ankle dorsiflexion limitations, poor alignment of posture, and impaired balance [2,7,8].

Suggested treatments for ITW vary, but the necessity and effectiveness of the treatments are controversial. The recommended approaches to overcome ITW include observation, special training procedures, muscle stretching, orthotic therapy, supportive footwear therapy, serial casting, intramuscular botulinum toxin type A (BTX-A) injection, and finally, surgical heel-cord lengthening [1,3,4,9]. Williams et al. [10] proposed a Toe Walking Tool, an online questionnaire to encourage the users to distinguish between ITW and toe walking associated with medical conditions. Their approach was found to be a valid and reliable tool for the diagnosis but does not serve as an immediate treatment to fix toe walking. In [9], stretching exercises and ankle-foot-orthoses are useful to keep adequate ankle dorsiflexion, and BTX-A reduces the development of plantar flexion torque. Engström et al. [11] explored the effectiveness of BTX-A with 24 months follow-up, but they concluded that injecting BTX-A did not significantly decrease toe walking. Davies et al. [12] studied the geology of ITW and the long-term effects of conservative therapy on gait performance. They concluded there was a reduction in toe walking severity in the active treatment group with casting. However, several studies [3,13] report that conservative treatments do not have any lasting effect on the toe walking, and even after surgical treatment, the failure rate is over 30% [4]. More promising analyses and interventions of ITW still need to be developed and validated.

Variability of gait parameters has been an indicator of health, such as Parkinson's disease [14], cardiovascular disease [15], fall detection [16], and cognitive decline [17]. Gait analysis has been used to monitor patient progress in orthopedics and rehabilitation [18]. A gait cycle (or stride events) contains a stance phase (initial contact, loading response, mid stance, terminal stance, and pre-swing) and a swing phase (initial swing, mid-swing, and terminal swing) [18]. Information about human locomotion includes quantitative measures (i.e., length, speed, and angle) of step, stride, stance, and swing. The traditional clinical assessments to analyze gait parameters rely on subjective or semi-subjective scales [18]. Subjective gait assessment tools, such as the Gait Abnormality Rating Scale [19], Four Square Step Test [20], and Functional Gait Assessment [21], are more likely to have observer variations which affect the accuracy of diagnosis [18]. Objective measurement to characterize human gait is obtainable through advancements in technology, including instrumented walking mats, treadmills, and motion capture systems [15]. These instruments are often expensive, difficult to use, and require a clinical setting to be installed and measured.

The development of wearable sensors and wireless communication encourages remote monitoring of human movements in natural settings. Wearable sensors can be attached to different body locations, such as the foot, waist, chest, wrist, or head [18]. Numerous wearable sensors have been used for the gait analysis: accelerometers, gyroscopic sensors, magnetometers, force sensors, extensometers, goniometers, active markers, and electromyography [15]. A low-power and short-range wireless medium, such as Bluetooth, ZigBee, ANT, Near Field Communications (NFC), are also available for body sensor networks [22]. Recent remote health monitoring systems [17,18,23] utilize a smartphone as a network hub or processing gateway for massive amounts of sensor data. The remote health monitoring system, which is low-cost, portable, and pervasive, enables a new healthcare era.

A real-time assessment system enables real-time intervention. Because ITW is a habitual or behavioral activity among healthy children, behavior change techniques (BCTs) [24] may motivate them to put their heels down. Based on control theory [25], designing a system to record walking activities to compare the daily number of toe strikes and heel strikes can bring positive outcomes to the individuals with ITW. The remote assessment system can prompt a specific goal setting (i.e., achieving more heel strikes) and provide an intuitive interface to review the goals compared to the recordings. These children may not need conservative or surgical treatments with high-cost clinical visits to overcome ITW. The system with wearable sensors can detect continuous toe walking and give just-in-time adaptive intervention (JITAI).

We introduce a remote toe walking monitoring system, GAIToe (**G**ait **A**nalysis utilizing an **I**nertial measurement unit (IMU) for **Toe** walking detection and intervention). The GAIToe uses a single IMU in an insole to detect physical activities such as toe walking, heel-toe walking, standing on toe, normal standing, sitting on toe (sitting heel raises), and normal sitting. It also provides real-time biofeedback with two types of vibrations: a short vibration for 3, 6, or 9 consecutive toe contacts and a long vibration for ten consecutive toe contacts on the ground. The long vibration can be turned off with a heel strike. The sensor data of GAIToe are transmitted to the developed Android application via Bluetooth Low Energy (BLE). The Android application stores the recordings in the cloud-based database and presents the number of toe steps and normal heel-toe steps. Our system affords a portable, non-invasive, low-cost, power-efficient, easy-to-use, and quantitative assessment. Using this system is expected to have positive impact on the population with ITW.

The remainder of the paper is structured as follows. Section 2 explores the related works on utilizing wearable sensors for gait analysis. Section 3 discusses the system specification of the GAIToe, including hardware implementation, power consumption, mobile app development, and the activity recognition algorithm. Section 4 presents the experiments and preliminary evaluation of GAIToe. Finally, we propose our future research direction in Sect. 5 and conclude in Sect. 6.

2   Related Works

Multiple wearable sensors have been proposed to provide information about human locomotion and activity recognition. Liu *et al.* [26] developed a wearable system to detect gait phases using multiple inertial sensors of gyroscopes and accelerometers. The sensor units are attached to the leg segments (the foot, shank, and thigh) using straps. Since many sensors' usability and appearance on the body regions are not practical, several studies have embedded sensors in the shoe or insole. Xu *et al.* [27] proposed a smart insole to compute gait parameters with 48 pressure sensors, a 3-axis accelerometer, a 3-axis gyroscope, and a 3-axis compass. Lin *et al.* [28] presented a smart insole that measures plantar pressure with an array of piezoelectric sensors and movement information with inertial sensors. Both studies developed smartphone software for data processing and real-time computing. Sazonov *et al.* [29] utilized five force-sensitive resistors (FSRs) placed on an insole and a 3-axis accelerometer positioned on the back of the shoes. Their sensor system recognized human body posture and activity by employing support vector machines (SVMs). Hegde *et al.* [30] proposed a pediatric smart shoe system for remote activity (sitting, standing, and walking) detection. They placed five FSRs and an accelerometer on the insole and mounted other electronics in the back of the shoes. Carbonaro *et al.* [31] achieved the detection of the gait phases (heel-strike, stance, heel-off, and swing) utilizing two FSRs located on the heel and forefoot and an accelerometer embedded in the forefoot, interfacing with a smartphone through Wi-Fi connection. All of these works are useful to track human locomotion and walking status. However, their complicated systems and algorithms are not designed specifically for toe walking detection and interventions.

Our proposed platform, GAIToe, detects different walking, sitting, and standing behaviors by integrating a single IMU in an insole. We selected an IMU because the shoes' acceleration data were sufficient to identify different gait patterns based on the literature and our experiments. The system costs less than $80.00 before the cost-saving of mass production. The sensor unit is not exposed and does not deform the exterior design of regular shoes. Furthermore, our activity recognition algorithm does not require complex sensor fusion algorithms because we use a single IMU on each insole. The computation of activity recognition is executed onboard; therefore, the portable sensing unit can give real-time feedback without requiring a connection to the server or the other devices for the determination. The developed Android application also provides visual feedback and serves as a data logger. Our platform motivates individuals with ITW to change their walking patterns with continuous remote monitoring in non-clinical settings.

3   GAIToe System Specification

GAIToe is composed of two main components: a shoe sensor unit and a linked smartphone application (Fig. 2). The sensor unit is designed to measure the foot movements using an IMU. It is mounted into an insole to be easily inserted into any running shoes. We programmed the sensor unit with a machine learning-based activity recognition algorithm for the real-time toe walking detection and feedback. The readings of the sensor unit are transmitted to an Android application via Bluetooth. The Android application stores the recordings in the cloud-based database. It also displays toe walking and heel-to-toe walking results for the individuals with ITW in order to review their daily walking patterns.

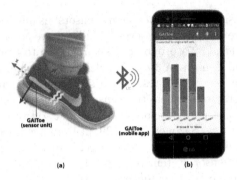

(a)   (b)

Fig. 1. Components of the system: (a) a sensor unit mounted on the insole and (b) a linked smartphone application. A sensor unit of the GAIToe, utilizing an IMU, detects toe walking and vibrates onboard. It transmits data to the connected smartphone application via Bluetooth.

3.1 Hardware Implementation

We investigated available wearable sensors, wireless data transmission modules, programmable controllers, and rechargeable batteries with small dimensions to develop remote monitoring and real-time intervention systems for habitual toe walkers in natural settings. Our hardware implementation goal was to maximize the utilization of currently available and affordable devices in order to reduce the expense of our custom-designed system.

With all these considerations, Adafruit Feather M0 Bluefruit LE (Adafruit Industries, New York, NY, adafruit.com) [32] development board was chosen. It has an ATSAMD21G18 ARM Cortex M0 processor with up to 48 MHz operating frequency, 32 KB SRAM memory, and 256 KB FLASH. Adafruit Feather provides Bluetooth Low Energy (BLE), low-power, 2.4 GHz spectrum wireless protocol. The Bluefruit LE module (nRF51822) uses the standard Nordic universal asynchronous receiver-transmitter (UART) RX/TX connection profile and enables transmitting data back and forth from an iOS or Android device. Adafruit Feather has a JST connector for 3.7 V Lithium-Polymer (Lipo) or Lithium-Ion (LiIon) battery. We selected an 800 mAh Lipo rechargeable battery as the power supply and connected a slider switch to control it. The built-in micro-USB port on the board allows us to program the microcontroller, as well as automatically switch between USB power and charging the connected Lipo battery at 100 mA. Several indicator LEDs provide the board's status, such as a red LED for power, a blue LED for BLE connection, and a yellow LED for charging. The board's dimension is 51 mm × 23 mm × 8 mm, reasonably small for any wearable device.

GAIToe is equipped with an MPU-9250 motion tracking device (9 degrees of freedom IMU). It is a multi-chip module consisting of a 3-axis accelerometer, a 3-axis gyroscope, and a 3-axis magnetometer (AK8963). The accelerometer has a measurement range of up to ±16 g and sensitivity up to 16, 384 LSB/g. The gyroscope has a range of ±2000°/s and sensitivity up to 131 LSB/deg/sec. The

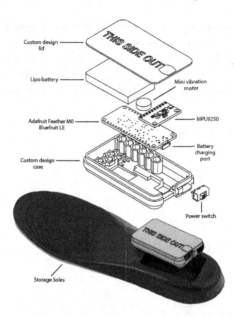

Fig. 2. Circuit components in a GAIToe sensor unit. The custom-designed 40 mm × 72 mm × 14 mm case is mounted on the storage soles and includes all the circuitry, such as an Adafruit Feather board, an IMU, a mini vibration motor, a Lipo battery, and a slide switch.

magnetometer's full-scale range is ±4800 μT, and the sensitivity is 0.6 μT/LSB. Each sensor outputs digitized values through three 16-bit analog-to-digital converters (ADCs). An MPU-9250 communicates with the Adafruit feather board via I²C bus at 400 kHz. The IMU in the insole is located to contact the calcaneus, the heel bone on the hindfoot, as can be seen in Fig. 1a. It captures the shoe acceleration, angular velocity, and magnetic north.

A mini vibration motor is connected to the Adafruit Feather board to provide real-time biofeedback. When the user is continuously toe walking or consistently standing and sitting on the toe (sitting heel raises), the GAIToe sensor unit produces vibration. Following three, six, and nine consecutive toe contacts (walking, standing, or sitting) on the ground, the GAIToe sensor unit generates 1-s vibration. Following ten consecutive toe contacts, it generates 30-s vibration. The long vibration can be turned off with a heel strike. This vibration generation protocol was defined in consultation with orthopedic surgeons and physical therapists as what would successfully arouse the user's attention regarding toe walking and motivate more heel strikes.

Storage soles [33], insoles with a container space at the bottom, satisfied our need to house the shoe sensor unit and to insert it into any running shoes. Storage soles are made from flexible polyurethane (PU) foam, so they are waterproof and easily trimmed for nearly any shoe size. We designed a case and lid to house the circuitry components and fit them into the storage soles. The case and lid are made by a 3D printer using polylactic acid (PLA), a common plastic filament material. The empty space in the case is filled with hexagons to endure the pressure of human body weight. The custom-designed 40 mm × 72 mm × 14 mm case includes all the circuitry (Fig. 2), such as an Adafruit Feather board, an IMU, a mini vibration motor, a lipo battery, and a slide switch.

3.2 Power Consumption

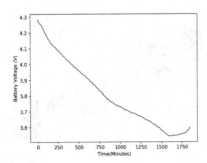

Fig. 3. Battery characteristics of GAIToe sensor unit. A Lipo battery discharge curve with continuous vibrations

The power efficiency of the system is crucial to monitor the foot activity and give continuous real-time intervention. We attempted to emulate a worst-case usage scenario, continuous toe sitting, including a series of vibrations and a transmission rate at 20 Hz. A typical Lipo battery maintains around 3.7 V for much of the battery life, then decreases in voltage just before the circuitry cuts it off. In our experiment, the battery almost consistently discharged the voltage and stayed at the minimum voltage of 3.545 V for 30 min. Interestingly, the battery increased the voltage up to 3.6 V before it turned off (Fig. 3). We figured out that the system lasts 1,845 min (30.75 h) under continuous operation (Fig. 3). Our system fits in clinical settings as well as continuous, pervasive monitoring in naturalistic settings. It requires getting charged every day and does not run out of charge during activities in a day.

3.3 Android Application Development

Our sensor unit is implemented to compute activity detection on the board but does not have a data logging component. We could add data storage, like an SD card, in the unit, but that would require an extra step of transferring data to monitor daily walking patterns. Due to the recent advancements in mobile technologies, smartphones are commonly used as a communication hub in the remote monitoring systems [28,31,34]. We developed an Android app (Fig. 1b) to achieve wireless data transmission, collecting data from our sensor unit via

Bluetooth, and storing the data in the cloud-based database via the Internet. We focused on a design with minimal user interaction.

The Android application includes a specific Bluetooth connection protocol to connect to the GAIToe sensor unit automatically. When the app is launched, it starts to scan and connect to the BLE module using the pre-stored MAC address. When the Bluetooth connection is stable, the UART serial communication between the BLE module and the Android device begins. If the UART service fails within 20 s, the app automatically terminates the BLE connection and scans the BLE module again. The Bluetooth connection can be reset manually by pressing the (three-dot) Connect button on the top right corner of the screen (Fig. 1b). The Bluetooth icon next to the Connect button indicates BLE connection status in four colors: disconnection in red, scanning phase in orange, stable connection with UART in white, and failed UART service in black. The average time for the Bluetooth connection was 5.242 s in an experiment with the LG Phoenix 4 smartphone (which has an Android 7.1.2 Nougat operating system and 1.4 GHz Quad-Core Qualcomm Snapdragon processor). The GAIToe sensor unit transmits the IMU's raw signals, the detected activities, and the generated vibration feedback to the connected app with 20 Hz.

The developed app provides an intuitive visualization of the daily walking pattern. Our app calculates an accumulated number of steps based on the received types of activity from the sensor unit. A stacked bar chart displays the number of toe steps in red bars and the number of heel-to-toe steps in green bars (Fig. 1b). The previous six days' step counts are shown on the first 6 bars while the real-time step counts are shown on the rightmost bar. The app saves the collected data into the cloud-based database every five minutes.

3.4   Activity Recognition Algorithm

In order to achieve the objective of providing a real-time system, we concentrated on developing the activity recognition algorithm on the microcontroller. Wearable IMU signals are sensitive to small foot movements, and the activities cannot be determined by a threshold-based algorithm. Tree-based machine learning models allowed us to achieve high classification accuracy with the IMU signals.

To train the activity classification model, we first collected activity data from 14 healthy subjects recruited from the university community. The subjects were asked to wear our study shoes with sizes vary from youth's size 6 to women's size 11. Then, they performed 200 strides of heel-toe walking and toe walking, as well as 2 min of sitting and standing. We made use of our Android application with an added functionality to save the activity label and the subject ID along with the sensor data in the database.

We extract features from the IMU data to feed the classifier. The magnitude of the 3-axis of accelerometer, gyroscope, and magnetometer is computed using Eq. 1.

$$A_i = \sqrt{x_i{}^2 + y_i{}^2 + z_i{}^2} \tag{1}$$

Where i is the index of the signal; and x_i, y_i, and z_i are the three-axis of vectors. A low-pass filter [35] is applied to the vectors of the accelerometer. We derive the roll and pitch angles from the acceleration data [35]. The tilt angles [36] of the 3-axis of each sensor are also calculated.

To train supervised machine learning classification algorithms on our time series data, we process the data by dividing it into windows of 10 data points. Then, according to Eqs. 2 and 3, the mean and standard deviation of each window are extracted as a feature.

$$WindowAverage_t = \frac{\sum_{i=1}^{n} x_i}{n} \tag{2}$$

Where x_i is a signal reading with index i and n is the size of the window which here is assumed to be 10.

$$WindowStandardDeviation_t = (\frac{\sum_{i=1}^{n}(x_i - WindowAverage_t)^2}{n-1})^{\frac{1}{2}} \tag{3}$$

We selected an extra-trees classifier from Scikit-Learn [37], which had the highest cross-validation (CV) result among other classifiers. This classifier predicts the class by implementing a meta estimator that fits randomized decision trees with sub-samples [37]. Using an extra-trees classifier, we ran the training data with various estimators (1 to 100) and maximum depths (1 to 20). Figure 4 demonstrates the cross-validation scores achieved from examining these estimators and maximum depths. Considering the limited flash memory (program space) on the Arduino-compatible microcontroller and analyzing Fig. 4, the best 10-fold cross-validation (88%) was achieved by setting the estimator to 25 and maximum depth to 8.

To remove the irrelevant features from our classification model, we ran tree-based feature selection [37]. Acceleration pitch and tilt angle mean, gyroscope magnitude mean, and standard deviation of gyroscope raw signal values are the most significant features among the others in our training model. The precision, recall, and F1-score of each label (normal walk, toe walk, normal sit/stand, and toe sit/stand) are reported in Fig. 5. According to Fig. 5, the normal sit/stand label has the highest precision and lowest recall; however, the toe walk label holds the lowest precision and highest recall. All four classes have roughly the same f-1 score.

Further, the leave one subject out cross-validation of the extra-trees with 25 estimators and maximum depth of 8 is 86%. In order to compute the leave one subject out cross-validation, for each subject, we train the classifier on the data collected from the other subjects, and then we test the classifier on the remaining subject's data. Therefore, we make sure that the training and test data are subject-independent.

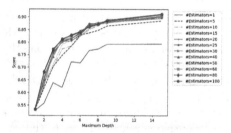

Fig. 4. The extra-trees classification cross validation scores using a various numbers of estimators and maximum depths. Running extra-tree classifier on training data using a various number of estimators (ranging from 1 to 100) and maximum depths (ranging from 1 to 20). The cross-validation score resulted from each run is reported. Then, considering our hardware limitations, the best estimator and maximum depth are selected.

After coming up with the classification model, if activity is determined as normal or toe walking, then the steps counting procedure takes place. Regarding the gait cycle, the forefoot is off the ground during the swing phase, which happens once for each step. Having this in mind and computing peak signals of all the features mentioned earlier, we conclude that nonconsecutive peak signals of gyroscope 3-axis magnitude in window size equal to 10 are an accurate estimation of step counts. To this end, for each window identified as walking, the signal retaining a higher value than the window average is classified as a peak of the window.

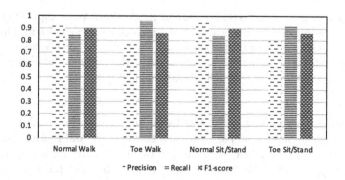

Fig. 5. Precision, recall, and F1-score of all labels. The precision, recall, and F1-score of all classes when running extra-tree classifier on training data with estimator and maximum depth equal to 25 and 8, respectively. The F1-score of all the labels are roughly the same.

Taking into account various walking paces, consecutive peak points are considered as a single step. Figure 6 elaborates an example of the steps count procedure in 2 consecutive windows of size 10. In Fig. 6, among the first 10 consecutive values of gyroscope magnitudes, the 1st, 5th, 6th, 7th, and 9th values are higher than the average of the window. Due to the sequence of 5th, 6th, and 7th signals; signals that indexed as 6 and 7 are not labeled as a step. Accordingly, static windows of gyroscope magnitude signals are processed one after another. As an example of handling consecutive windows in Fig. 6, the last signal (index 9) of the first window is marked as a step. Incidentally, the first signal (index 10) of the second window carries a higher value than the mean signal values of the second window. Since the first window's last signal and the second window's first signal are consecutive, the last one is not perceived as a step. We programmed the microcontroller by integrating the exported C code of the extra trees classification model and step counts procedure.

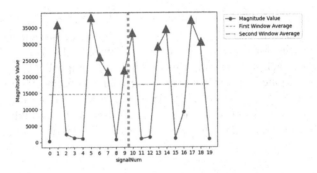

Fig. 6. Steps count peak detection in successive windows. An example of step counts procedure through 2 consecutive windows of gyroscope 3-axis magnitude. The windows are separated with a grey vertical dashed line. The average of each window is depicted using a horizontal dashed line. The signal values with a higher value than the average of their window are marked with red triangles. (Color figure online)

As previously explained in the Hardware Implementation section, to prevent users from continuous toe steps, after each third, sixth, and ninth successive toe step detection, a short vibration with a duration of a second is generated, and there is a long vibration with a duration of 30 s after the tenth successive toe step detection. The long vibration is halted as soon as a heel strike is perceived. Regarding the heel strikes detection in our machine learning classification, any activity labeled as normal heel-to-toe walking, normal sitting, and normal standing is remarked a heel strike. The same intervention procedure takes place for being on the toes while sitting or standing. In this case, every 400 ms of sitting or standing on toes is taken in to account as a step unit for the procedure. Giving these vibrations can notify the individuals about their continuous toe steps and remind them to put their heel down.

4   Experiments

Ten healthy adults (between the ages of 21 and 44) volunteered to try our GAIToe in their running shoes for the preliminary system evaluation. They attempted six activities: 100 strides of toe walking, 100 strides of normal heel-to-toe walking, 2-minute toe standing, 2-minute normal standing, 2-minute toe sitting, and 2-minute normal sitting. We instructed the participants to perform these activities correctly and then supervised them in order to obtain clear data. Subjects were asked to walk at a comfortable pace on level ground. This data was synchronized with the connected Android device.

Figure 7 shows the results of our activity detection and steps count algorithm evaluation. There is no incorrectly detected toe step during normal heel-to-toe walking of all subjects. However, within 100 toe steps of some subjects, there are incorrectly detected normal steps varying between 2 to 9. The average accuracy of normal heel-to-toe step counts and toe step counts are 93.6% $\pm$ 3.2 and 84.1% $\pm$ 5, respectively.

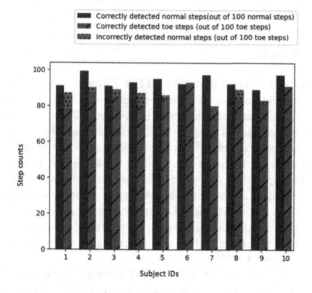

Fig. 7. Number of steps detected per subject. Results of steps detection and count. The solid blue bars show the number of correctly detected heel-toe normal steps through 100 heel-toe normal steps. There is no incorrectly detected toe step within normal walking. The green hatched (//) bars are the number of correctly detected toe steps out of 100 toe steps. Finally, the red dotted bars show the number of incorrectly detected heel-toe steps through 100 toe steps.

To evaluate our vibration protocol performance, we kept a record of the short and long vibrations while subjects walked for 100 toe steps. Table 1 reports the number of short and long vibrations within correctly detected toe steps. Any incorrectly detected normal steps through 100 toe strikes disrupt our vibration policy. If all the correctly counted toe steps were consecutive and all the packages have been delivered via the board to phone Bluetooth communication, the number of expected short and long vibrations would be what is recorded in the last two rows of Table 1.

Table 1. Number of short and long vibrations within 100 toe steps per subject. Reporting the number of short and long vibrations along with the number of correctly detected toe steps out of 100 toe steps. The expected number of short and long vibrations based on the correctly detected toe steps are reported in the last two rows as well.

Subject ID	1	2	3	4	5	6	7	8	9	10
Number of correctly detected toe steps	78	87	85	79	84	93	80	83	81	91
Number of short vibrations	20	27	26	23	25	28	24	25	24	28
Number of long vibrations	6	8	7	6	8	9	8	8	8	9
Expected number of short vibrations	23	26	25	24	25	28	24	25	24	27
Expected number of long vibrations	7	8	8	7	8	9	8	8	8	9

5   Future Work

We are actively recruiting children with ITW through the local children's hospital. We will provide a pair of Nike Revolution 5 FlyEase running shoes to the subjects as a constant measurement instrument. These running shoes have a wraparound zipper that is convenient for inserting and removing our insoles. The subjects and their parents will be educated to alter the insole based on their shoe size and install our software on a study Android device to monitor subjects' daily toe and heel-toe steps. We will ask the subjects to run our Android app in the background and wear the waist bag with the smartphone while trying our shoes. They will be responsible for charging the system every day. The subjects will benefit from real-time feedback when they have a series of toe walking. We will examine our system's effectiveness and robustness through their behavior change regarding their walking patterns.

Since IMU signals are sensitive to a small movement, we can reduce the signals' noise by applying various signal processing techniques. We will enhance our detection algorithm to reduce possible false positives in different situations, such as taking a stair or walking on the uphill path. The repeated usage and pressure on the circuitry container can break our custom-built sensor unit because it is located underneath the hindfoot, a place within the foot region that holds high pressure values [38]. We need to validate the robustness and durability of the system through a long-term assessment. Moreover, we can extend our study to identify the IMU-based gait parameters of ITW. GAIToe may enable orthopedic experts and researchers to investigate the detailed gait parameters and foot movements of ITW in natural settings. It may become an assistive tool to develop a more effective intervention technique.

6   Conclusion

In this paper, we proposed GAIToe, a remote-monitoring system for activity recognition and improving walking patterns of individuals with habitual toe walking. GAIToe provides a wearable, portable, energy-efficient, and low-cost platform for pervasively monitoring walking patterns in daily life. Our sensor unit, utilizing an IMU, is designed to be inserted into any running shoe. The proposed activity recognition algorithm is developed to identify different activities and give real-time biofeedback. It has been validated through an experiment on ten healthy subjects. The connected Android app provides visual feedback regarding walking patterns. Our system has the potential to improve an individual's walking behavior. Furthermore, their orthopedist can monitor the patient's progress remotely.

References

1. Williams, C.M., Tinley, P., Curtin, M.: Idiopathic toe walking and sensory processing dysfunction. J. Foot Ankle Res. **3**(1), 1–6 (2010)
2. Ruzbarsky, J.J., Scher, D., Dodwell, E.: Toe walking: causes, epidemiology, assessment, and treatment. Curr. Opin. Pediatr. **28**(1):40–46 (2016)
3. Stricker, S.J., Angulo, S.J.: Idiopathic toe walking: a comparison of treatment methods. J. Pediatr. Orthop. **18**(3), 289–293 (1998)
4. Hirsch, G., Wagner, B.: The natural history of idiopathic toe-walking: a long-term follow-up of fourteen conservatively treated children. Acta Paediatr. **93**(2), 196–199 (2004)
5. Shulman, L.H., Sala, D.A., Chu, M.L.Y., McCaul, P.R., Sandler, B.J.: Developmental implications of idiopathic toe walking. J. Pediatr. **130**(4), 541–546 (1997)
6. Engelbert, R., Gorter, J.W., Uiterwaal, C., van de Putte, E., Helders, P.: Idiopathic toe-walking in children, adolescents and young adults: a matter of local or generalised stiffness? BMC Musculoskelet. Disord. **12**(1), 61 (2011)
7. Goldstein, M., Harper, D.C.: Management of cerebral palsy: equinus gait. Dev. Med. Child Neurol. **43**(8), 563–569 (2001)
8. van den Hecke, A., Malghem, C., Renders, A., Detrembleur, C., Palumbo, S., Lejeune, T.M.: Mechanical work, energetic cost, and gait efficiency in children with cerebral palsy. J. Pediatr. Orthop. **27**(6), 643–647 (2007)
9. Williams, C.M., Pacey, V., de Bakker, P.B., Caserta, A.J., Gray, K., Engelbert, R.H.H.: Interventions for idiopathic toe walking. Cochrane Database Syst. Rev. **2016**(10), (2016)
10. Williams, C.M., Tinley, P., Curtin, M.: The toe walking tool: a novel method for assessing idiopathic toe walking children. Gait Posture **32**(4), 508–511 (2010)
11. Sätilä, H., Beilmann, A., Olsén, P., Helander, H., Eskelinen, M., Huhtala, H.: Does botulinum toxin a treatment enhance the walking pattern in idiopathic toe-walking? Neuropediatrics **47**(03), 162–168 (2016)
12. Davies, K., Black, A., Hunt, M., Holsti, L.: Long-term gait outcomes following conservative management of idiopathic toe walking. Gait Posture **62**, 214–219 (2018)
13. Eastwood, D.M., Menelaus, M.B., Dickens, D.R., Broughton, N.S., Cole, W.G.: Idiopathic toe-walking: does treatment alter the natural history? J. Pediatr. Orthop. Part B **9**(1), 47–49 (2000)

14. Zhang, H., et al.: Towards passive medication adherence monitoring of Parkinson's disease using smartphone-based gait assessment. In: Proceedings of the ACM on Interactive, Mobile, Wearable and Ubiquitous Technologies, vol. 3, 1–23 (2019)
15. Muro-De-La-Herran, A., Garcia-Zapirain, B., Mendez-Zorrilla, A.: Gait analysis methods: An overview of wearable and non-wearable systems, highlighting clinical applications. Sensors 14(2), 3362–3394 (2014)
16. Bianchi, V., Grossi, F., Matrella, G., De Munari, I., Ciampolini, P.: Fall detection and gait analysis in a smart home environment. Gerontechnology 7(2), 73 (2008)
17. Gwak, M., Woo, E., Sarrafzadeh, M.: The role of accelerometer and gyroscope sensors in identification of mild cognitive impairment. In 2018 IEEE Global Conference on Signal and Information Processing (GlobalSIP), pp. 434–438. IEEE (2018)
18. Anwary, A.R., Yu, H., Vassallo, M.: Optimal foot location for placing wearable IMU sensors and automatic feature extraction for gait analysis. IEEE Sens. J. 18(6), 2555–2567 (2018)
19. Brach, J.S., Van Swearingen, J.M.: Physical impairment and disability: relationship to performance of activities of daily living in community-dwelling older men. Phys. Therapy 82(8), 752–761 (2002)
20. Duncan, R.P., Earhart, C.M.: Four square step test performance in people with Parkinson disease. J. Neurol. Phys. Therapy 37(1), 2–8 (2013)
21. Wrisley, D.M., Kumar, N.A.: Functional gait assessment: concurrent, discriminative, and predictive validity in community-dwelling older adults. Phys. Therapy 90(5), 761–773 (2010)
22. Majumder, S., Mondal, T., Jamal Deen, M.: Wearable sensors for remote health monitoring. Sensors 17(1), 130 (2017)
23. Can, Y.S., Arnrich, B., Ersoy, C.: Stress detection in daily life scenarios using smart phones and wearable sensors: a survey. J. Biomed. Inform. 92,103139 (2019)
24. Abraham, C., Michie, S.: A taxonomy of behavior change techniques used in interventions. Health Psychol. 27(3), 379 (2008)
25. Carver, C.S., Scheier, M.F.: Control theory: a useful conceptual framework for personality-social, clinical, and health psychology. Psychol. Bull. 92(1), 111 (1982)
26. Liu, T., Inoue, Y., Shibata, K.: Development of a wearable sensor system for quantitative gait analysis. Measurement 42(7), 978–988 (2009)
27. Xu, W., Huang, M.-C., Amini, N., Liu, J.J., He, L., Sarrafzadeh, M.: Smart insole: a wearable system for gait analysis. In: Proceedings of the 5th International Conference on Pervasive Technologies Related to Assistive Environments, pp. 1–4 (2012)
28. Feng, L., Aosen, W., Yan, Y., Tomita Machiko, R., Wenyao, X.: Smart insole: a wearable sensor device for unobtrusive gait monitoring in daily life. IEEE Trans. Ind. Inform. 12(6), 2281–2291 (2016)
29. Sazonov, E.S., Fulk, G., Hill, J., Schutz, Y., Browning, R.: Monitoring of posture allocations and activities by a shoe-based wearable sensor. IEEE Trans. Biomed. Eng. 58(4), 983–990 (2010)
30. Hegde, N., et al.: The pediatric smartshoe: wearable sensor system for ambulatory monitoring of physical activity and gait. IEEE Trans. Neural Syst. Rehabil. Eng. 26(2), 477–486 (2017)
31. Carbonaro, N., Lorussi, F., Tognetti, A.: Assessment of a smart sensing shoe for gait phase detection in level walking. Electronics 5(4), 78 (2016)
32. lady ada. Adafruit feather M0 Bluefruit LE. Accessed 20 Jan 2019
33. CoolThings: Storage soles shoe insoles with hidden storage, January 2019
34. Gwak, M., et al.: Extra: exercise tracking and analysis platform for remote-monitoring of knee rehabilitation. In: 2019 IEEE 16th International Conference on Wearable and Implantable Body Sensor Networks (BSN), pp. 1–4. IEEE (2019)

35. AnilM3. Arduino IMU: Pitch & roll from an accelerometer, January 2019
36. Accelerometers
37. Pedregosa, F., et al.: Scikit-learn: machine learning in Python. J. Mach. Learn. Res. **12**, 2825–2830 (2011)
38. Mazur, F., et al.: Plantar pressure changes in hindfoot relief devices of different designs. J. Exp. Orthop. **6**(1), 1–8 (2019). https://doi.org/10.1186/s40634-019-0173-9

Applied Computing – Life and Medical Sciences

Prediction of Conversion to Alzheimer's Disease Using 3D-DWT and PCA

Li Yew Aow Yong[1]([✉]) [ID], Mohd Shafry Mohd Rahim[1] [ID], and Chi Wee Tan[2] [ID]

[1] School of Computing, Faculty of Engineering, Universiti Teknologi Malaysia,
81310 Johor Bahru, Johor, Malaysia
ylyaow2@live.utm.my

[2] Faculty of Computing and Information Technology, Tunku Abdul Rahman University College,
Kuala Lumpur, Malaysia

Abstract. Alzheimer' Disease (AD) is the most common form of dementia worldwide. Structural Magnetic Resonance Imaging (sMRI) is the supportive tool for the diagnosis of this disease. Even, it can be used to predict the conversion of the disease from the mild cognitive impairment (MCI) to AD stage. Nevertheless, the 3D image produced by sMRI is high dimensional data, which raises the risk of overfitting in the classification model. For this reason, the combination of Discrete Wavelet Transform (DWT) and Principal Component Analysis (PCA) was proposed as the feature extraction techniques to reduce the dimensional and extract significant features concurrently. The issues of DWT are the selection of level of decomposition and wavelet filter to decompose the image. In order to deal with these issues, a series of experiments were conducted to find the suitable parameters. By using 2D-DWT, spatial information of 3D data cannot be captured. The connection between the slices is neglected. Hence, 3D-DWT has been adopted instead of 2D-DWT in this paper. In the classification step, Support Vector Machine (SVM) was used as the classifier to predict the conversion of normal control (NC) and stable MCI (SMCI) to progressive MCI (PMCI) and AD for datasets collected up to 2 years before the progression. The dataset used in this paper was collected from Alzheimer's Disease Neuroimaging Initiative (ADNI) database. In the validation, the proposed method outperformed the other methods by attaining 79%, 79%, 82% and 82% in accuracy for the datasets collected at different time points, which were 1% to 4% higher than the model adopted 2D-DWT and PCA.

Keywords: Alzheimer's Disease · Structural MRI · DWT · PCA

1 Introduction

Alzheimer's Disease (AD) is a degenerative brain sickness which eventually leads to death due to complications [1]. The death rate of AD was increased 146% from year of 2000 to 2018, while other diseases such as heart's disease had decreased in United States. The patient suffers AD experiences cognitive and behavioral impairment such as memory loss, difficulty in thinking and reasoning, and personality change. Hence, it

© ICST Institute for Computer Sciences, Social Informatics and Telecommunications Engineering 2022
Published by Springer Nature Switzerland AG 2022. All Rights Reserved
S. Spinsante et al. (Eds.): HealthyIoT 2021, LNICST 432, pp. 199–213, 2022.
https://doi.org/10.1007/978-3-030-99197-5_16

requires a lot of time and money in taking care the patient suffers AD. In light of the AD facts and figures, it is becoming extremely difficult to ignore the existence of AD. The early prediction of the conversion to AD is getting more attention to provide a more comprehensive treatment to the patient. Also, it prepares the heart of the caregiver to provide emotional support and daily support to the patient.

There have been a number of longitudinal studies involving Structural Magnetic Resonance Imaging (sMRI) that have been reported to be the supportive tool in AD diagnosis [2]. MRI is a non-invasive brain imaging technique [3], therefore, it is more preferable compared to other brain imaging techniques as well. SMRI reveals the internal structure of the brain. Hence, the atrophy of the brain can be detected through examining the 3D image produced from the device. The longitudinal study of MRI images of a patient provides more information to the doctor on the formation of the disease [4]. On the other hand, a single scan also allows the doctor to identify the existence of AD with the help of brain imaging and neuropsychological tests.

There are several stages in the development of AD. The healthy patients are categorized as normal control (NC), the patients suffer mild cognitive impairment (MCI) but they do not convert to AD after a period of observation are categorized as stable mild cognitive impairment (SMCI), the patients suffer MCI and they converts to AD after a period of observation are categorized as progressive MCI (PMCI), and AD refers to the patients are having AD at the baseline scan. The prediction of the conversion to AD in computer-aided diagnosis involves classifying the different stages of the disease, especially on segregating PMCI from SMCI to prescribe the right medicine to the patient.

Nevertheless, the brain image produced from sMRI is high dimensional data. Each 3D image contains millions of features, and it causes overfitting. Hence, feature extraction is an important procedure before classification. This paper has proposed Discrete Wavelet Transform (DWT) and Principal Component Analysis (PCA) to perform feature extraction. Some of the researchers had adopted 2D-DWT instead of 3D-DWT in their studies. However, 2D-DWT faces the issue of losing spatial information. It does not consider the connection between the slices of 3D image during the data compression [5]. Besides, the main challenges of DWT are selecting suitable wavelet and decomposition level. Different kinds of datasets require different parameter selection. Hence, 3D-DWT was adopted in this paper. In order to deal with the parameter selection issue, experiments were conducted to examine the performance of different parameters towards the AD classification.

The main contribution of this paper is to identify the best parameters for 3D-DWT on the AD image. It ensures the extracted features increase the accuracy of classification. The results in the comparison demonstrate that the proposed method has achieved better performance compared to other models. The rest of the paper is organized as follows: Sect. 2 presents the prior study, Sect. 3 describes the proposed method, Sect. 4 discusses the implementation and evaluation, Sect. 5 provides the results and discussion, and Sect. 6 draws the conclusion for this paper.

2   Prior Study

The selection of feature extraction approaches in AD classification is based on the features used in the studies. The Gray Level Co-occurrence Matrix (GLCM) was widely used in extracting texture features of the brain image [6–8]. Tooba Altaf et al. [6] computed the texture features such as entropy, contrast, correlation and homogeneity by applying GLCM in each slice of the 3D MR image. Then, the average of the features was obtained to form a feature vector for each MR image. Besides, the authors also adopted scale invariant feature transform, local binary pattern and histogram of oriented gradient to extract texture features. Besides extracting texture features, Arpita Raut and Vipul Dalal [7] also extracted shape and area features by using moment invariants. A total of 13 features were extracted from the image. C.V. Dolph et al. [8] had extracted the features such as volume, surface area and cortical thickness by using FreeSurfer software. The texture feature was extracted through the proposed novel fractal texture feature extraction, which was the combination of fractal dimension and GLCM.

Apart from the methods aforementioned, voxel-based morphometry (VBM) is also another approach to compare the differences between the groups in voxel-wise [9]. The VBM approach proved that grey matter alternation is consistent with the neuropsychological test. It also found that the healthy patient who faces cognitive impairment in future has reduced grey matter density compared to the patient who remains normal cognitive [10]. Thus, the voxel-wise comparison was also widely used in AD classification. The VBM analysis can be conducted by using different software, such as FSL-VBM and Statistic Parameter Mapping (SPM) [10–12]. The number of VBM features is usually higher than the samples, therefore, Principal Component Analysis (PCA) and Partial Least Square (PLS) were commonly used to further extract and reduce the features [13, 14]. Both techniques were always compared, and PLS outperformed PCA in most studies. L. Khedher et al. [14] drew the graphs to compare the classification result by using different numbers of features. It showed that the number of features is the key to determine the classification results for both techniques.

Besides, it is noticed that the combination of PCA with DWT has improved the classification result. Yudong Zhang et al. [15] proposed 3D-DWT to extract the wavelet coefficients of the image. Then, the volume descriptors were calculated through the subbands obtained from each level of decomposition. PCA was used to find the uncorrelated features. This study showed that 3D-DWT outperformed 2D-DWT by preserving the spatial information of 3D images. Luis Javier Herrera et al. [5] performed 2D-DWT and PCA in their study. However, the results showed that the combination with PCA decreased the classification result. This might be due to the number of features selected for PCA having impacts on the results. Apart from that, both studies adopted DWT with different wavelets. In view of the controversial claims, this study aims to give a comprehensive view on the selection of suitable wavelet and level of decomposition for AD classification. However, it is impossible to compare the results with the previous studies because different features and different population studies have been used in the study. By using different scope, it brings great impact on the classification results. This study has conducted a voxel-wise comparison between the groups without using any descriptors. As a result, this study validated the proposed method by comparing the classification results of different parameters, and the evaluation of different models was done on the collected datasets.

There were several classifiers that have been used by the research in AD classification. Support Vector Machine (SVM) was one of the widely used classifiers [13, 14, 16]. It involved linear SVM, kernel SVM or other variations of SVM. It has been proved that it is powerful in dealing with the AD classification by achieving good results, which were 80% and above accuracy in most of the cases. SVM was popularly used in binary classification, in contrast, deep learning approach especially convolutional neural network was commonly used for multiclass classification [8, 17]. However, parameter tuning is the main concern of deep learning approaches because there is lack of guidelines on determining the layers in between [18, 19]. A trial-and-error process is required to determine the number of hidden layers and neurons. Deep learning approach is treated as an one stop solution for AD classification, which has included feature extraction in the layers. Therefore, this paper chose to adopt SVM as classifier to perform binary classification.

3   Proposed Method

In this section, the proposed feature extraction techniques of this paper are presented. The AD classification scheme involved three steps, which were pre-processing, feature extraction and classification (see Fig. 1). The pre-processing was done through Computational Anatomy Toolbox (CAT12) software to segment the gray matter (GM) tissue with default parameters. The images were normalized to Montreal Neurological Institute (MNI) space by using Diffeomorphic Anatomic Registration Through Exponentiated Lie algebra algorithm (DARTEL) template to allow further analysis. The 3D images which contained the segmented GM tissue were transformed to $121 \times 145 \times 121$ voxels. After this, the 3D images underwent feature extraction by using 3D-DWT and PCA. The low dimensional data obtained from the feature extraction was the input of linear SVM classifier. The details of feature extraction and classification methods are described in the following sub-sections.

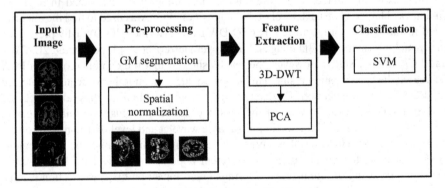

Fig. 1. Alzheimer's disease classification scheme

3.1   3D-Discrete Wavelet Transform

DWT is a time-frequency analysis which is used for data denoising or data compression by choosing appropriate frequency bands. In image processing, the image is treated as signal and edges, which provide the frequency information to the algorithm [20]. The image is passed into a low pass filter and a high pass filter to find the image details. DWT compresses the data, at the same time, it extracts the significant features in the down sampling process. In order to decide the level of decomposition and wavelet for 3D-DWT, experiments were done to examine the results by using different parameters. The results are reported in Sect. 5. At last, 3-level 3D-DWT with Haar wavelet was adopted in this paper as the first step of feature extraction.

The 3-level 3D-DWT indicates that it involves three times decomposition at the approximation coefficients obtained from previous level of decomposition, and it takes part of three axes of the data. Figure 2 shows the diagram of 3-level 3D-DWT, where L refers to low pass filter, H refers to high pass filter, and downward arrow refers to down sampling process.

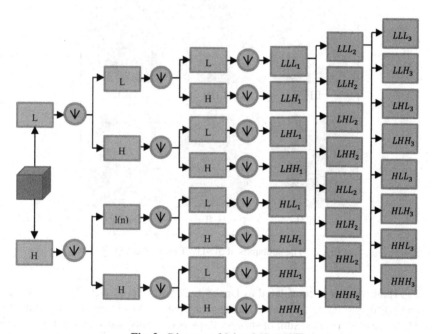

Fig. 2. Diagram of 3-level 3D-DWT

The 3D-DWT can be done through passing the 3D image in row, column and slice direction to the filter. Therefore, it produces 8 subbands named as LLL, LLH, LHL, LHH, HLL, HLH, HHL, HHH. The subband LLH is obtained through passing the image to low pass filter along x-axis, low pass filter along y-axis and high pass filter along z-axis. The other subbands also can be interpreted through this concept. Figure 3 provides the examples of the subbands obtained from 1-level 3D-DWT on the sagittal image. The subband LLL produces an approximation coefficient of the image, and it is used for further decomposition. On the other hand, the other subbands capture the detailed coefficients of the image by passing through a high pass filter in any of the direction.

The image is down sampled by 2, therefore, the size of the image in each dimension from each level of decomposition is half of the previous level.

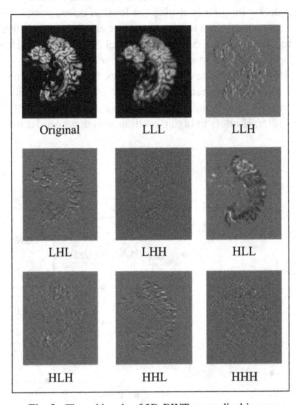

Fig. 3. The subbands of 3D-DWT on medical image

The Haar wavelet is considered as Daubechies 1 wavelet as well. It is the simplest wavelet but it is suitable for the AD images as compared to other wavelet filters [5]. The Haar wavelet takes the sum of successive pairs of pixels' values in each axis of the image, then multiplying it with the normalization constant, $1/\sqrt{2}$. This forms the 3D low pass filter matrix, LLL as shown in Eq. (1). The low pass filter in this paper had size of ($2 \times 2 \times 2$), which produced the coarser image by examining 8 pixels' values at a time until the whole image was decomposed. The subband LLL was used as the input of PCA. As a result, the 3-level 3D-DWT reduced the size of pre-processed image to 16 $\times$ 19 $\times$ 16 dimensions, which was 4,864 features.

$$LLL = \left[\left[\left[\frac{1}{2\sqrt{2}}\frac{1}{2\sqrt{2}}\right]\left[\frac{1}{2\sqrt{2}}\frac{1}{2\sqrt{2}}\right]\right]\left[\left[\frac{1}{2\sqrt{2}}\frac{1}{2\sqrt{2}}\right]\left[\frac{1}{2\sqrt{2}}\frac{1}{2\sqrt{2}}\right]\right]\right] \quad (1)$$

3.2 Principal Component Analysis

PCA is a linear transformation approach which projects the image data points to lower dimensional space. PCA finds the lines that maximize the variance of the data to obtain the minimal representation of the original image. The lines are called principal axes. Principal components are obtained through projecting the data points to the principal axes. The first principal component has the largest variance of the data, and the variance goes down to the last principal component.

Eigen-decomposition is the classical way to find the direction and magnitude to project the data. However, it might face accuracy loss due to eigenvalues are sensitive to perturbations in some matrices [21]. Any changes of the matrices will lead to great changes in eigenvalues. Therefore, singular value decomposition (SVD) was used as a replacement for eigen-decomposition in this paper due to its numerically stable in computation.

The 3D image from DWT was transformed to 1D long feature vector, and all the training set samples were stacked together to form the input of PCA. The input data has undergone mean-centring to decompose to $U\Sigma V^T$. The columns of U are called left singular vector, which contains the unit vectors, the diagonal of Σ are singular values, which contains the sum of projection lengths, and the columns of V are called singular vector, which contains the projection directions. The rank of mean-centring data, X_{mean} is $r = \min(m, n)$ to gain non-zero singular values, where m is number of samples and n is the number of dimensions of each sample. Consequently, the full SVD can be simplified to economy SVD as illustrated in Fig. 4.

The equation for economy SVD is derived as Eq. (2), where U is m-by-m matrix, $\widehat{\Sigma}$ is m-by-m matrix and $\widehat{V}^T$ is m-by-n matrix. Then, the covariance matrix can be computed from Eq. (3). By obtaining the covariance matrix through SVD, the projection of the input data was done through multiplying with $\widehat{V}^T$ to obtain the low-dimensional uncorrelated data.

$$X_{mean} = U\Sigma V^T = U\begin{bmatrix} \widehat{\Sigma} \\ 0 \end{bmatrix} V^T = U\widehat{\Sigma}\left[\widehat{V}^T \widehat{V}^{\perp T}\right] \tag{2}$$

$$X_{mean}{}^T X_{mean} = V\Sigma U^T U\Sigma V^T = \widehat{V}\widehat{\Sigma}^2\widehat{V}^T \tag{3}$$

Each principal component refers to the transformed feature for classification. The dataset used in this paper had 160 samples for training set, as a result, the number of features after PCA was 159. All the features were kept in this paper to avoid eliminating the useful features, since low variance principal components also contributed to segregate the classification groups.

3.3 Support Vector Machine

In this paper, the only classifier was soft margin linear SVM. The soft margin SVM can deal with the situation where there are outliers fall in the areas belong to different groups. This makes it more suitable compared to hard margin SVM when the classifier deals with real-world data because the data might not distribute linearly. SVM finds the

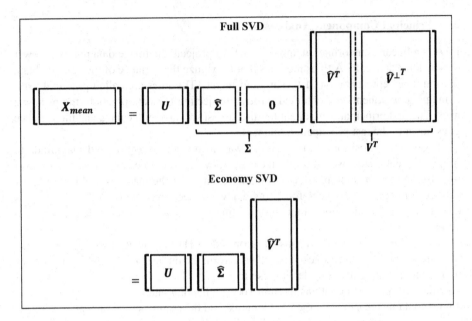

Fig. 4. Full and economy SVD

hyperplane which separates different groups. It needs to fulfill two requirements, which are having the largest distance with the nearest data and minimizing the classification loss. The hyperplane is found through following Eq. 4 subjects to Eq. 5, where the w denotes vector, x denotes features or variables of the image, b denotes the biased term, y denotes the predicted label, ξ refers to the distance between outlier and the correct margin, and n refers to the total number of features.

$$\min_{w,b} \frac{1}{2}\|w\|^2 + \sum_{i=1}^{n} \xi_i \qquad (4)$$

$$y_i\left(w^T x_i + b\right) \geq 1 - \xi_i \qquad (5)$$

4   Implementation and Evaluation

Based on the proposed method in Sect. 3, the experiments were conducted to identify suitable wavelet and level of decomposition for 3D-DWT. The dataset, evaluation method and evaluation metric are described in this section.

4.1   Dataset Acquisition

The datasets were collected from the Alzheimer's Disease Neuroimaging Initiative (ADNI) database. The ADNI was launched in 2003 as a public-private partnership, led by Principal Investigator Michael W. Weiner, MD. The primary goal of ADNI has been to test whether serial magnetic resonance imaging (MRI), positron emission tomography (PET), other biological markers, and clinical and neuropsychological assessment can be combined to measure the progression of mild cognitive impairment (MCI) and early Alzheimer's disease (AD). For up-to-date information, see www.adni-info.org.

The datasets were collected at different time points, which were 24 months before stable diagnosis, 18 months before stable diagnosis, 12 months before stable diagnosis and at the stable diagnosis time point. Each dataset consisted of 50 NC, 50 SMCI, 50 PMCI and 50 AD. The dataset collected during stable diagnosis time point refers to the patients who had ended the observation periods which lasted for 24 months. The subjects in the SMCI category refer to the patients remaining in MCI state at the end of the observation, while the subjects in the PMCI category refer to the patients convert to AD even though they had been diagnosed as MCI during baseline scan.

All the MR images obtained were pre-processed T1-weighted MR images, which had undergone 3D gradient inhomogeneity correction and B1 non-uniformity correction [22, 23]. After that, the images were further processed by using CAT12 as mentioned in Sect. 3. This paper conducted binary classification, which divided the different categories into two groups. The NC and SMCI was grouped together as (NC + SMCI) to represent the healthier patient, and the PMCI and AD was grouped together as (PMCI + AD) to represent the sick patient. Hence, the prediction on the conversion can be done by comparing the binary groups.

4.2 K-Fold Cross-Validation

Cross-validation allows assessing the model without bias. A 5-fold cross-validation was employed in this paper to perform out-of-sample assessment on the model. The assessment was done on the independent set. The 5-fold cross-validation divided the datasets to five subsets randomly. The training set was built with four subsets and the validation set was constructed with the last subset. This procedure was repeated for 5 times, and the different classification groups were divided equally in each cross-validation partition. All datasets were divided into training set and validation set before PCA instead of classification. This is because PCA is a machine learning approach which requires a training set to find the projection direction first. Then, the validation set will be projected based on the training set's projection direction.

4.3 Evaluation Metric

The aim of this paper is to improve the accuracy of AD classification. Therefore, the evaluation metric used in this paper was mean accuracy from the cross-validation. After obtaining the accuracies from each cross-validation, the average of the accuracies was calculated to be the overall result. Accuracy gauges the ability of the model in correctly predicting the conversion of the disease in this paper context [24]. It calculates the number of correct predictions from the total number of predictions. Accuracy is derived from the confusion matrix, which calculates the true positive (TP), true negative (TN), false positive (FP) and false negative (FN) in the predictions. The confusion matrix is demonstrated in Table 1, and the accuracy is calculated by using Eq. 6.

$$Accuracy = (TP + TN)/(TP + FP + TN + FN) \tag{6}$$

Table 1. Confusion matrix for AD classification

		Predicted class	
		(PMCI + AD)	(NC + SMCI)
Actual class	(PMCI + AD)	TP	FN
	(NC + SMCI)	FP	TN

TP = the number of (PMCI + AD) subjects is identified as (PMCI + AD).
TN = the number of (NC + SMCI) subjects is correctly identified as (NC + SMCI).
FP = the number of (NC + SMCI) subjects is identified as (PMCI + AD).
FN = the number of (PMCI + AD) subjects is identified as (NC + SMCI).

5   Results and Discussion

The purpose of conducting the experiments was to identify the suitable wavelet filter and level of decomposition for AD classification. Therefore, the mean accuracy from the cross-validation was the measurement in these experiments. The experiments had compared different popular wavelets, which included Haar, Daubechies (Db) 2, Db4, Symlet (Sym) 2 and Sym4 with different levels of decomposition of 3D-DWT on the four datasets collected at different time points. The initial decomposition was set to 2-level. The criteria to stop the increment of the decomposition level was the dropping of the mean accuracy.

Table 2 shows the 2-level 3D-DWT with different wavelets. The results revealed that the selection of wavelets had a great impact on classification results especially on the dataset collected at time points of 24 months and 18 months before stable diagnosis. It is challenging to classify the datasets collected at the earlier time points. The mean accuracies of the datasets collected at time points of 24 months and 18 months before stable diagnosis were always lower than the datasets collected at later time points. Despite this, Sym4 wavelet achieved the best results compared to other wavelets in 2-level 3D-DWT.

Table 3 shows that 3-level 3D-DWT by using Sym4 wavelet and Haar wavelet achieved higher mean accuracies compared to 2-level 3D-DWT with Sym4 wavelet at all time points except the dataset collected at time point of 18 months before stable diagnosis. The lowest mean accuracy of 3-level 3D-DWT with Haar wavelet on different datasets was 1% higher compared to Sym4 wavelet. Nevertheless, the Sym4 wavelet achieved 1% higher in the highest accuracy.

Table 2. The classification results with 2-level 3D-DWT and PCA

	24 m before stable diagnosis	18 m before stable diagnosis	12 m before stable diagnosis	Stable diagnosis time point
Haar	0.77	0.78	0.80	0.81
Db2	0.78	0.77	0.80	0.81
Db4	0.76	0.80	0.81	0.81
Sym2	0.78	0.77	0.80	0.81
Sym4	0.77	0.80	0.81	0.81

Table 3. The classification results with 3-level 3D-DWT and PCA

	24 m before stable diagnosis	18 m before stable diagnosis	12 m before stable diagnosis	Stable diagnosis time point
Haar	0.79	0.79	0.82	0.82
Db2	0.78	0.78	0.82	0.80
Db4	0.76	0.77	0.83	0.80
Sym2	0.78	0.78	0.82	0.80
Sym4	0.80	0.78	0.81	0.83

Table 4 shows that the classification dropped significantly in the 4-level 3D-DWT on most of the wavelets except Db4. However, the overall classification results of 4-level 3D-DWT by using Db4 did not show improvement compared to 3-level 3D-DWT by using Haar or Sym4 wavelet. Therefore, the experiment was stopped at 4-level 3D-DWT. The possible reason for dropping the classification result is the significant features for AD classification will be omitted when it is up to 4-level decomposition. DWT is a fine-to-coarse method, it is a trade-off relationship between compression ratio and the accuracy, due to the details of the image are being eliminated in each level of decomposition.

Table 4. The classification results with 4-level 3D-DWT and PCA

	24 m before stable diagnosis	18 m before stable diagnosis	12 m before stable diagnosis	Stable diagnosis time point
Haar	0.72	0.76	0.77	0.82
Db2	0.75	0.78	0.77	0.80
Db4	0.80	0.77	0.80	0.82
Sym2	0.75	0.78	0.77	0.80
Sym4	0.76	0.76	0.75	0.78

In view of the results, this paper proposes to use 3-level 3D-DWT with Haar wavelet. Even though Sym4 can achieve higher results in certain datasets, but it is more important to increase the lowest accuracy obtained from different datasets to ensure more cases can be predicted correctly. The output of 3-level 3D-DWT on the image is demonstrated in Fig. 5. The image is given with the axes to show the size of the image in pixels after each decomposition level. As aforementioned, the size of the output image in each dimension is half of the original size. Hence, the output of first level of decomposition was $(61 \times 73 \times 61)$, as the original size was $(121 \times 145 \times 121)$. The down-sampling process was repeated in the second and third level of decomposition. Eventually, there was 4,864 features left after DWT. The number of features of the image was further reduced by using PCA. There were 159 features to be fed into classifier.

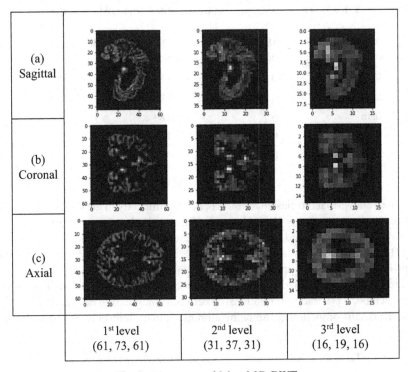

Fig. 5. The output of 3-level 3D-DWT

It is impossible to benchmark with the literature provided in this paper due to different features and different datasets were used in the studies. Therefore, a comparison of different models was conducted with the same datasets are demonstrated in Table 5. The first model adopted PCA and SVM, the second model applied 2D-DWT, PCA and SVM, and the proposed model implemented 3D-DWT, PCA and SVM. It is noticed that applying 2D-DWT and PCA as the feature extraction techniques did not increase the mean accuracy, but it dropped the results on the datasets collected at time point of 18 months and 12 months before stable diagnosis. On the other hand, 3D-DWT obtained

2%–4% higher compared to use PCA and SVM only on most of the datasets except the dataset collected at time point of 18 months before stable diagnosis. Even though there is an exception, but 3D-DWT still gives a promising result on most of the datasets. The results also indicated that 3D-DWT compresses the image more accurately compared to 2D-DWT. The significant features can be captured from 3D-DWT.

Table 5. The comparison of different models

	24 m before stable diagnosis	18 m before stable diagnosis	12 m before stable diagnosis	Stable diagnosis time point
PCA	0.75	0.80	0.79	0.80
2D-DWT + PCA	0.76	0.78	0.78	0.80
Proposed	0.79	0.79	0.82	0.82

6 Conclusion

This paper has proposed to apply 3-level 3D-DWT with Haar wavelet and PCA as the feature extraction for AD classification. There were different wavelet families used in previous study, this paper has clarified that the most suitable wavelet is Haar wavelet. Besides, the maximum level of decomposition shall set to 3 because the significant features will be eliminated along the decomposition process. By using the suitable wavelet and level of decomposition, 3-level 3D-DWT and PCA improved the classification result in predicting the conversion to AD.

It is worth to note that all principal components obtained from PCA was used in this paper. Feature selection was not included in this model to avoid the high sensitivity issue, due to different number of features gives high impact on the classification result. Nevertheless, it is necessary to examine the scheme of AD classification to further improve the results. The additional data such as age, gender and neuropsychological test can be included to boost the classification result. Without surprise, the prediction of the conversion to AD is more challenging on the datasets collected in the earlier stage of the disease compared to the datasets collected at time point which are near to stable diagnosis. Therefore, more attention shall be focused on the early diagnosis of the disease to provide better treatment to the patients. The future work can be done on designing the AD classification scheme to enlarge the difference between the classification group, which shall give a more distinguishable boundary for the classifier.

Acknowledgements. The authors would like to thank Universiti Teknologi Malaysia (UTM) for supporting this research. The authors also acknowledge that the data used in this study was obtained from the Alzheimer's Disease Neuroimaging Initiative (ADNI) database (adni.loni.usc.edu). As such, the investigators within the ADNI contributed to the design and implementation of ADNI and/or provided data but did not participate in analysis or writing of this report. A complete listing of ADNI investigators can be found at: http://adni.loni.usc.edu/wp-content/uploads/how_to_apply/ADNI_Acknowledgement_List.pdf.

The data was funded by ADNI (National Institutes of Health Grant U01 AG024904) and DOD ADNI (Department of Defense award number W81XWH-12-2-0012). ADNI is funded by the National Institute on Aging, the National Institute of Biomedical Imaging and Bioengineering, and through generous contributions from the following: AbbVie, Alzheimer's Association; Alzheimer's Drug Discovery Foundation; Araclon Biotech; BioClinica, Inc.; Biogen; Bristol-Myers Squibb Company; CereSpir, Inc.; Cogstate; Eisai Inc.; Elan Pharmaceuticals, Inc.; Eli Lilly and Company; EuroImmun; F. Hoffmann-la Roche Ltd and its affiliated company Genentech, Inc.; Fujirebio; GE Healthcare; IXICO Ltd.; Janssen Alzheimer Immunotherapy Research & Development, LLC.; Johnson & Johnson Pharmaceutical Research & Development LLC.; Lumosity; Lundbeck; Merck & Co., Inc.; Meso Scale Diagnostics, LLC.; NeuroRx Research; Neurotrack Technologies; Novartis Pharmaceuticals Corporation; Pfizer Inc.; Piramal Imaging; Servier; Takeda Pharmaceutical Company; and Transition Therapeutics. The Canadian Institutes of Health Research is providing funds to support ADNI clinical sites in Canada. Private sector contributions are facilitated by the Foundation for the National Institutes of Health (www.fnih.org). The grantee organization is the Northern California Institute for Research and Education, and the Study is coordinated by the Alzheimer's Therapeutic Research Institute at the University of Southern California. ADNI data are disseminated by the Laboratory for Neuro Imaging at the University of Southern California.

References

1. Alzheimer's Association: 2020 Alzheimer's disease facts and figures. Alzheimer's & Dementia **16**(3), 391–460 (2020)
2. Dubois, B., et al.: Research criteria for the diagnosis of Alzheimer's disease: revising the NINCDS-ADRDA criteria. Lancet Neurol. **6**(8), 734–736 (2007)
3. Soucy, J.-P., et al.: Clinical applications of neuroimaging in patients with Alzheimer's disease: a review from the fourth Canadian consensus conference on the diagnosis and treatment of demantia. Alzheimer's Res. Therapy **5**(1), 1 (2013)
4. Ledig, C., Schuh, A., Guerrero, R., Heckemann, R.A., Rueckert, D.: Structural brain imaging in Alzheimer's disease and mild cognitive impairment: biomarker analysis and shared morphometry database. Sci. Rep. **8**(1), 1–6 (2018)
5. Herrera, L.J., Rojas, I., Pomares, H., Guillén, A., Valenzuela, O., Baños, O.: Classification of MRI images for Alzheimer's disease detection. In: 2013 International Conference on Social Computing, pp. 846–851 (2013)
6. Altaf, T., Anwar, S.M., Gul, N., Majeed, M.N., Majid, M.: Multi-class Alzheimer's disease classification using image and clinical features. Biomed. Signal. Process. Control **43**, 64–74 (2018)
7. Raut, A., Dalal, V.: A machine learning based approach for detection of Alzheimer's disease using analysis of hippocampus region from MRI Scan. In: IEEE International Conference on Computing Methodologies and Communication, pp. 236–242 (2017)
8. Dolph, C.V., Alam, M., Shboul, Z., Samad, M.D., Iftekharuddin, K.M.: Deep learning of texture and structural features for multiclass Alzheimer's disease classification. In: 2017 International Joint Conference on Neural Networks (IJCNN), pp. 2259–2266. IEEE (2017)
9. Margarida Matos A., Faria P., Patricio M.: Voxel-based morphometry analyses in Alzheimer's disease. In: 2013 IEEE 3rd Portuguese Meeting in Bioengineering (ENBENG), pp. 1–4. IEEE (2013)
10. Tondelli, M., Wilcock, G.K., Nichelli, P., De Jager, C.A., Jenkinson, M., Zamboni, G.: Structural MRI changes detectable up to ten years before clinical Alzheimer's disease. Neurobiol. Aging **33**(4), 825-e25 (2012)

11. Beheshti, I., Demirel, H.: Probability distribution function-based classification of structural MRI for the detection of Alzheimer's disease. Comput. Biol. Med. **64**, 208–216 (2015)

12. Wang, W.-Y., et al.: Voxel-based meta-analysis of grey matter changes in Alzheimer's disease. Transl. Neurodegener. **4**(1), 1–9 (2015)

13. Salvatore, C., Cerasa, A., Castiglioni, I.: MRI Characterizes the progressive course of AD and predicts conversion to Alzheimer's dementia 24 months before probable diagnosis. Front. Aging. Neurosci. **10**, 135 (2018)

14. Khedher, L., Ramírez, J., Górriz, J.M., Brahim, A., Segovia, F.: Early diagnosis of Alzheimer's disease based on partial least squares, principal component analysis and support vector machine using segmented MRI images. Neurocomputing **151**, 139–150 (2015)

15. Zhang, Y., Wang, S., Phillips, P., Dong, Z., Ji, G., Yang, J.: Detection of Alzheimer's disease and mild cognitive impairment based on structural volumetric MR images using 3D-DWT and WTA-KSVM trained by PSOTVAC. Biomed. Signal Proces. Control **21**, 58–73 (2015)

16. Jongkreangkrai, C., Vichianin, Y., Tocharoenchai, C., Arimura, H.: Computer-aided classification of Alzheimer's disease based on support vector machine with combination of cerebral image features in MRI. J. Phys. Conf. Ser. **694**, 012036 (2016)

17. Fulton, V.L., Dolezel, D., Harrop, J., Yan, Y., Fulton, C.P.: Classification of Alzheimer's Disease with and without Imagery using gradient boosted machines and ResNet-50. Brain Sci. **9**(9), 212 (2019)

18. Munteanu, C.R., et al.: Classification of mild cognitive impairment and Alzheimer's disease with machine-learning techniques using 1H magnetic resonance spectroscopy data. Expert. Syst. App. **42**(15–16), 6205–6214 (2015)

19. Ebrahimighahnavieh, M.A., Luo, S., Chiong, R.: Deep learning to detect Alzheimer's disease from neuroimaging: a systematic literature review. Comput. Methods Programs. Biomed. **187**, 105242 (2020)

20. Ejaz, K., et al.: Segmentation method for pathological brain tumor and accurate detection using MRI. Int. J. Adv. Comput. Sci. App. **9**(8), 394–401 (2018)

21. Moler, C.B.: Eigenvalues and singular values. In: Numerical Computing with Matlab, pp. 269–305. Society for Industrial and Applied Mathematics (2004)

22. Jovicich, J., et al.: Reliability in multi-site structural MRI studies: effects of gradient non-linearity correction on phantom and human data. NeuroImage **30**(2), 436–443 (2006)

23. Jack, C.R., et al.: The Alzheimer's disease neuroimaging initiative (ADNI): MRI methods. J. Magn. Reason. Imaging. **27**(4), 685–691 (2008)

24. Baratloo, A., Hosseini, M., Negida, A., El Ashal, G.: Part 1: simple definition and calculation of accuracy sensitivity and specificity. Emergency **3**(2), 48–49 (2015)

DIY Wrist-Worn Device for Physiological Monitoring: Metrological Evaluation at Different Band Tightening Levels

Angelica Poli[1], Gloria Cosoli[2(✉)], Lorenzo Verdenelli[2],
Francesco Scardulla[3], Leonardo D'Acquisto[3], Susanna Spinsante[1],
and Lorenzo Scalise[2]

[1] Department of Information Engineering, Università Politecnica delle Marche, 60131 Ancona, Italy
{a.poli,s.spinsante}@pm.univpm.it
[2] Department of Industrial Engineering and Mathematical Sciences, Università Politecnica delle Marche, 60131 Ancona, Italy
{g.cosoli,l.verdenelli,l.scalise}@staff.univpm.it
[3] Department of Engineering, Università degli Studi di Palermo, 90128 Palermo, Italy
{francesco.scardulla,leonardo.dacquisto}@unipa.it

Abstract. Wearable devices are currently employed in several application fields, especially in the healthcare context, thanks to the advent of IoT technology in the global market. However, there are few studies focused on the reliability of collected data depending on the best wearing conditions, e.g. the band tightness in the case of wrist-worn devices, necessary to optimise the quality of the measured data. The aim of this study is to evaluate the variability of heart rate (HR) and tightening force data measured with a *Do-It-Yourself* (DIY) wrist-worn device, considering three different band tightening levels: loose, medium and tight. Results show that the increasing tightening levels produce an increasing tightening force, as expected; interestingly, the coefficient of variation is minimum (i.e., 0.16%) when the band tightening level is medium.

Keywords: Photoplethysmographic sensor · Wearable device · Health monitoring · Reliability · Metrological characterization · Data variability

1 Introduction

Wearable devices are currently employed in many different application fields, such as individual activity monitoring, rehabilitation and fitness/sport performance assessment [31,37], sleep quality evaluation [22,36], health tracking of elderly people in Ambient Assisted Living (AAL) scenario - also to improve their Quality of Life (QoL) - [2,3,35], monitoring of physiological parameters for the treatment and diagnosis of different diseases [20], early diagnosis of viruses

© ICST Institute for Computer Sciences, Social Informatics and Telecommunications Engineering 2022
Published by Springer Nature Switzerland AG 2022. All Rights Reserved
S. Spinsante et al. (Eds.): HealthyIoT 2021, LNICST 432, pp. 214–229, 2022.
https://doi.org/10.1007/978-3-030-99197-5_17

symptoms (e.g., in COVID-19 pandemic [10,33]), Industry 4.0 [9], etc. Hence, wearable technologies are catching on in the healthcare context, thanks to multiple reasons: smartwatch-like devices are in fact user-friendly, relatively low-cost (with respect to standard equipment for the monitoring of physiological parameters) and available in distinct forms, several cost and quality segments, capable to satisfy different customer types, also thanks to user-experience oriented design of these tools. Also miniaturised devices, promoting comfort and user-friendliness of such systems, are topics of interest for the current research [12]. Moreover, it is worthy to underline that nowadays a single device can provide many different physiological/activity-related parameters, such as heart rate (HR) [27], heart rate variability (HRV) [19], energy expenditure [17], blood oxygen saturation [4], respiratory rate [14], number of steps [8], walked distance, etc. [15,30]. An additional success of wearable devices is attributable to the possibility of remote health monitoring thanks to the fact that, with a proper Internet-of-Things (IoT) architecture, they are capable to connect with other devices and share individual data e.g. on a Cloud platform, making them remotely available and safely stored. This is particularly relevant in health monitoring applications, also to support the healthcare providers in decision-making processes [6]. On the other hand, there are aspects requiring particular attention when using the data gathered by wearable devices; in fact, such systems are capable to provide data 24 hours a day, seven days a week. This generates a huge amount of data, the so-called "big-data" [16], potentially useful to train Artificial Intelligence (AI) algorithms for different purposes: well-being assessment [7], personal comfort measurement [13,26], stress level quantification [21,23], just to cite some. However, privacy-related issues should be properly considered, managing these individual data fulfilling the national and international regulations [5]. On the other hand, the evaluation of accuracy and reliability of these smartwatches are aspects still needing a lot of research [11,24]. It is beyond doubt that the hardware characteristics of the device influence the quality of measurement results [28]; also the correct positioning is of utmost importance to collect reliable data. When wearing a smartwatch, the band tightness obviously influences the measurement results, since sensors are susceptible to the contact pressure with skin. In particular, the functioning of the photoplethysmographic (PPG) sensor, commonly used to acquire the signal related to cardiac activity (indeed, it measures the changes in the blood volume, caused by the pumping activity of the heart [25]), is generally based on a light emitting diode (LED) and a photodetector [34]; hence, the measured signal depends on the quantity and quality of light received by the photodetector after being emitted by the LED and having crossed the skin tissues. Given that PPG sensor is very prone to motion artefacts, it would be necessary to optimise its positioning in order to maximise the signal-to-noise ratio (SNR), while minimising the environmental light that can reach the photodetector, and maximising the capture of the light reflected/transmitted by the skin (depending on the type of the PPG sensor, which can be based on reflection or transmission, respectively [29]). In order to take these aspects into account, it is fundamental to guarantee an optimal contact between the PPG sensor and the subject's wrist skin, maintaining a constant and stable position during the whole daily activities. In fact, different tightness values determine a different vibration in wrist-worn devices, turning into a different signal quality. In particular, a loose band would make output data not reliable if compared to the reference electrocardiographic (ECG) signal [18]. However, to the best of the authors' knowledge, concerning the consumer wearable devices, neither manufacturers provide specific indications on the optimal band tightening level value that should be achieved in order to maximise the signal quality, nor data related to this type of investigation are available in literature. Therefore, it would be interesting to add this evaluation during the smartwatch design phase, in order to give customers indications useful to obtain reliable results. Some of the authors performed a study to identify the optimal contact pressure capable to optimise the accuracy in the measurement of HR, considering a chest-strap device as gold standard instrument [32]. In the present study, the authors have realised a prototype of wrist-worn device including both a PPG sensor and a load cell, in order to quantify the effect of different tightening levels of the band on the recorded signal, evaluating in particular its variability. Ten healthy volunteer subjects have been enrolled to collect data for the evaluation of the measurement repeatability, as well as the effect of different band tightening levels and, consequently, of different tightening force values on the measurement of the HR. The paper is organised as follows. Section 2 provides details on the wrist-worn device developed in this study, the signal acquisition methodology and the postprocessing of data. Section 3 reports and discusses the obtained results. Finally, Sect. 4 contains the authors' conclusions, with final considerations on the study and future work.

2   Materials and Methods

2.1   Wrist-Worn Acquisition Device

The PPG data were recorded by using a *Do-It-Yourself* (DIY) wrist-worn wearable device. The device consists of a PPG sensor (Keyestudio XD-58C Pulse Sensor, with a 515 nm green light LED), a button load cell (FX1901, Meas. Spec., Schaffhausen, Switzerland), an amplifier board HX711 and an Arduino ATmega2560 with a sampling rate of 9600 Hz as acquisition board. The assembled device is shown in Fig. 1, whereas the separate components in Fig. 2.

Concerning the employed sensors, the PPG sensor was fixed in place by means of glue on a custom 3D-printed watch case, whereas the load cell was placed on a 3D printed casing, in order to be held in position every time the wrist band is worn. The CAD models and the overall assembly with both the PPG and load cell sensors are shown in Fig. 3.

The wrist band support was connected to a 3D-printed load cell presser, as it can be seen in Fig. 4.

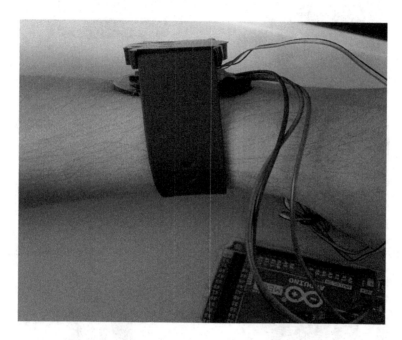

Fig. 1. Wrist-worn wearable device assembly.

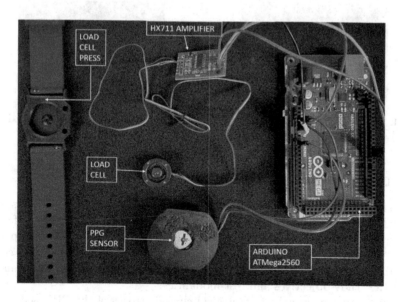

Fig. 2. Wrist-worn wearable device components.

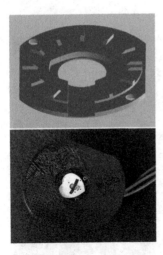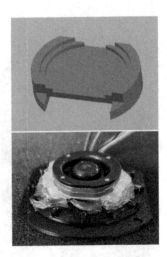

Fig. 3. CAD models and overall assembly of PPG (left) and load cell (right) casings.

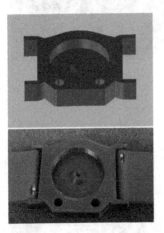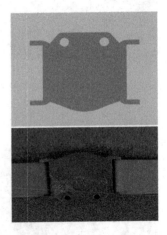

Fig. 4. 3D-printed load cell presser and wrist band assembled: front (left) and back (right) views.

2.2 Data Acquisition Protocol

Ten healthy subjects, 4 males and 6 females aged between 21 and 31 years, with a Body Mass Index (BMI) between 19 and 26 kg/m^2 and a wrist circumference between 14 and 19 cm, with a skin colour classification of Type II (Fitzpatrick scale), were involved in the experimental tests. Before starting the data collection, all the subjects signed an informed consent, providing adequate information about the study objectives and test modalities.

In order to evaluate the metrological characteristics of the PPG sensor, the participants were submitted to nine sessions: three repetitions, lasting 30 s per each, for the three levels of band tightness (i.e., *loose*, *medium* and *tight*). The band tightening levels were defined as shown in Table 1, according to the subject's wrist size. The wrist size was considered as the *loose* level (starting point), i.e. with the band length equal to the wrist circumference (L_0, tightening of 0.00 cm).

Table 1. Tightening levels of the band - (L_0 is the subject's wrist circumference)

Tightening level	Band length
Loose	L_0 - 0.00 cm
Medium	L_0 - 0.50 cm
Tight	L_0 - 1.00 cm

The DIY wrist-worn device was placed on the same wrist as the one where each of the subjects usually wears her/his watch (5 subjects on right wrist and 5 subjects on the left one). An automatic oscillometric digital blood pressure monitor was employed to collect subjects' data related to blood pressure (BP) and HR before starting the acquisitions; this device was positioned on the left arm, as generally recommended. Furthermore, the measurements were repeated after having changed the band tightness. In particular, the prototype wearable device worn at the *loose* level was tested according to the subject wrist circumference. After 30 s, the band was unfastened and then braced again to test the PPG measurement repeatability. The same procedure, repeated for three times, was adopted for the *medium* and *tight* levels, with +0.50 cm and +1.00 cm of band tightening, respectively. During the tests, participants were required to avoid hand and/or arm movements to reduce the motion artefacts potentially compromising the measurements. Moreover, data collected by using both the PPG sensor and the load cell were graphically displayed with the Telemetry software [1] to have a preliminary signals visual inspection. Indeed, data from the load cell helped to verify that the reached tightening level was comparable, over all the subjects, irrespective of the personal wrist circumference.

2.3 Data Processing

The data gathered with the DYI wrist-worn device were processed in MATLAB environment. At first, both PPG and load-cell signals were resampled at 1 kHz, by using the modified Akima piecewise cubic Hermite interpolation. Then, the signal peaks were searched for the computation of HR from PPG signal. Once the HR series were obtained, the statistical quantities were derived, namely the mean (μ), the standard deviation (σ) and the coefficient of variation (c_v, also known as relative standard deviation) computed as follows:

$$c_v = \sigma/\mu \tag{1}$$

Similarly, data collected through the load cell was processed in order to obtain the μ, the σ and the c_v during each acquisition, hence verifying that the band tightening system was effective and that the contact pressure levels among different subjects were compatible, as well as repeatable on the same subject. Histograms were plotted to describe the distribution of the measurement results; the number of bins (K) was computed by means of the Sturges' rule formula, as follows:

$$K = 1 + \frac{10}{3}log_{10}(N), \tag{2}$$

where N is the numerosity of the sample.

3   Results and Discussions

In this section, the authors report the results related to the intra-subject repeatability of both HR and tightening force data measured with the three different band tightening levels (i.e., *loose*, *medium* and *tight*), as well as the inter-subject variability. It is worthy to highlight that a high repeatability is desired for what concerns tightening force (in order to give recommendations on the optimal wearing conditions), whereas HR variability is mainly due to the individual physiological state. However, HR related variability should be rather low in short acquisitions and considering resting conditions.

3.1   BP and HR Data Measured with the Oscillometric Method

Before changing the band tightening level, both HR and BP data were measured on each subject, including the maximum and minimum pressure values (named systolic and diastolic, respectively) with the oscillometric method by means of an automatic digital blood pressure monitor. The related measurement accuracies are ± 3 mmHg, and $\pm 4\%$ of the reading, for BP and HR, respectively. Resulting data, along with the subject's wrist circumference (accuracy of ± 0.1 cm), are reported in Table 2.

3.2   Results from Wrist-Worn PPG Sensor and Load Cell

Concerning the tightening force values obtained from the load cell, it is possible to notice that the same band tightening level resulted in different tightening force values (see Fig. 5). This is probably due to the different subjects' wrist circumference and morphology (i.e., physiological diversity), which means a different contact condition between the band, consequently the load cell, and the skin. However, considering the whole test population along with all the acquired force signals, the variability (quantified with the standard deviation, St. dev.) among the subjects is quite low ($c_v < 1\%$, see Table 3).

Table 2. BP and HR values measured on the test population with the oscillometric method: results obtained in the test sessions performed with different band tightening levels.

Subject	Wrist circumference [cm]	Tightening level	Systolic BP [mmHg]	Diastolic BP [mmHg]	HR[bpm]
1	15.0	Loose	115	74	87
		Medium	103	65	85
		Tight	108	63	79
2	14.0	Loose	110	77	91
		Medium	112	71	76
		Tight	113	68	78
3	17.0	Loose	122	76	75
		Medium	117	70	78
		Tight	116	69	81
4	14.0	Loose	118	86	63
		Medium	121	90	62
		Tight	85	51	63
5	16.0	Loose	119	76	90
		Medium	114	69	90
		Tight	113	70	89
6	16.0	Loose	115	62	58
		Medium	140	78	71
		Tight	128	78	72
7	15.5	Loose	113	61	80
		Medium	105	68	80
		Tight	96	57	80
8	19.8	Loose	107	62	50
		Medium	115	61	52
		Tight	-	-	-
9	17.0	Loose	116	71	60
		Medium	111	72	64
		Tight	106	64	64
10	15.5	Loose	101	66	69
		Medium	103	57	73
		Tight	95	59	69

On the other hand, considering the variability within the same subject (i.e., intra-subject variability), higher standard deviation values are reported for some subjects with respect to others (e.g., subject no. 5). However, considering all the tightening levels, it is possible to observe a homogeneous increasing trend (from *loose* to *tight* level) for all the subjects, even if different absolute values of force are reported, as it can be seen in Fig. 5.

The force distributions related to the data acquired with different band tightening levels are reported in Fig. 6: the force distribution is unimodal (not normal), with a positive skew (i.e., the tail is on the right).

Table 3. Inter-subject variability related to tightening force values obtained from the load cell, with the three different tightening levels (i.e., *loose*, *medium* and *tight*).

Tightening level	Tightening force		
	Mean [N]	St. dev. [N]	c_v [%]
Loose	0.49	0.15	0.30
Medium	1.07	0.17	0.16
Tight	2.51	0.62	0.24

Table 4. Inter-subject variability related to HR obtained from PPG sensor, with the three different tightening levels (*loose*, *medium* and *tight*).

Tightening level	HR		
	Mean [bpm]	St. dev. [bpm]	c_v [%]
Loose	81	15	18
Medium	80	13	16
Tight	81	14	17

Regarding the inter-subject variability of PPG results, the values obtained with the three different band tightening levels are compatible (see Table 4), considering that HR parameter shows an intrinsic physiological variability, irrespective of the band tightness. Moreover, the distributions of HR values are approximately Gaussian-like, as it can be observed in Fig. 7.

However, it is worthy to underline that the device wearing conditions undoubtedly influence the quality of the acquired data and, consequently, the reliability of the measurement results.

In particular, the measured tightening force is different depending on the wearing conditions of the device. It is possible to see that the mean value increases with tightening level, as expected (see Table 3 and Fig. 5). However, the coefficient of variation shows a trend not coherent with the tightening level, suggesting that it is possible to obtain more stable results with a higher tightening level of the band. The lowest variation is obtainable with the medium tightening level (corresponding to a tightening of 0.50 cm with respect to the subject's wrist circumference).

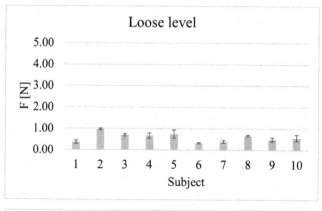

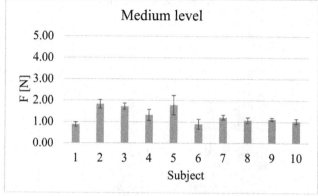

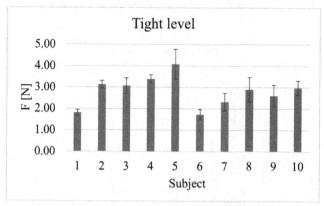

Fig. 5. Tightening force intervals (mean ± standard deviation) measured for *loose* (top), *medium* (centre) and *tight* (bottom) levels, for the whole population.

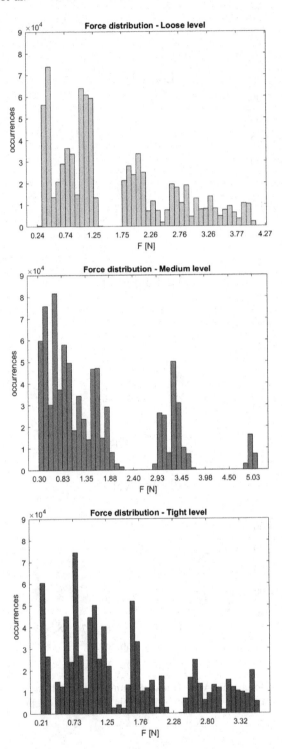

Fig. 6. Distribution of the measured tightening force in the tests with different tightening levels: *loose* (top), *medium* (centre) and *tight* (bottom), for the whole population.

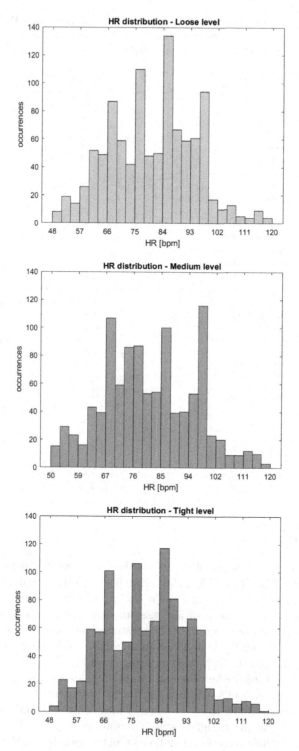

Fig. 7. Distribution of the measured HR in the tests with different tightening levels: *loose* (top), *medium* (centre) and *tight* (bottom), for the whole population.

Table 5. Intra-subject repeatability related to HR obtained from PPG signals and tightening force values measured from the DIY wrist-worn device, with the three different tightening levels (*loose*, *medium* and *tight*).

Subject	Tightening level	HR			Tightening force		
		Mean [bpm]	St. dev. [bpm]	c_V [%]	Mean [N]	St. dev. [N]	c_V [%]
1	Loose	74	10	14	0.37	0.08	0.21
	Medium	73	10	14	0.88	0.10	0.11
	Tight	71	7	10	1.81	0.14	0.08
2	Loose	99	6	6	0.97	0.03	0.04
	Medium	94	7	7	1.83	0.20	0.11
	Tight	98	10	10	3.13	0.18	0.06
3	Loose	82	6	7	0.70	0.05	0.07
	Medium	81	6	7	1.73	0.14	0.08
	Tight	87	6	6	3.07	0.36	0.12
4	Loose	81	11	13	0.67	0.12	0.18
	Medium	79	8	10	1.33	0.26	0.19
	Tight	77	7	9	3.39	0.20	0.06
5	Loose	68	10	14	0.75	0.19	0.25
	Medium	75	8	11	1.78	0.44	0.24
	Tight	68	6	10	4.08	0.69	0.17
6	Loose	90	4	4	0.33	0.03	0.10
	Medium	93	4	4	0.90	0.23	0.24
	Tight	94	4	4	1.73	0.23	0.13
7	Loose	73	6	8	0.40	0.07	0.18
	Medium	76	9	11	1.21	0.11	0.09
	Tight	80	8	10	2.32	0.41	0.17
8	Loose	91	9	10	0.67	0.04	0.05
	Medium	79	5	6	1.07	0.12	0.11
	Tight	81	8	9	2.90	0.57	0.19
9	Loose	70	8	11	0.50	0.09	0.18
	Medium	65	19	29	1.13	0.06	0.06
	Tight	70	23	32	2.61	0.50	0.19
10	Loose	68	5	7	0.57	0.15	0.26
	Medium	67	4	7	1.03	0.11	0.11
	Tight	67	7	11	2.98	0.33	0.11

4   Conclusion

In this study, the authors investigated whether and how different tightening levels of a wrist-worn band can affect the variability of the collected data (from PPG and load cell sensors) and, hence, the reliability of the measurement results. In particular, for each data acquisition session, three band tightening levels were considered: *loose*, *medium* and *tight*. The results show that, over all the subjects, the different tightening levels produce an increasing tightening force when passing from *loose* to *tight* through *medium* level; however, the coefficient of variation is minimum (i.e., 0.16%) when the band tightening level is *medium*. This is compliant also to the subject's comfort conditions in wearing the DIY wrist-worn wearable device, since the *tight* level sometimes causes discomfort, particularly in those subjects having a higher wrist circumference (i.e., >17 cm). However, further interesting investigations can be conducted focusing on the optimal band tightening in real life, when the subjects perform activities of daily living. This means to evaluate the reliability of the HR measurements at both rest and dynamic conditions; indeed, motion artefacts could be reasonably more significant during free-living conditions. According to our findings, the load cell could be avoided and replaced with a commercial watch wristband, used at different predefined tightening levels, starting from the subject's wrist circumference (i.e., *loose* level). Such replacement can be performed after a dedicated calibration of the different tightening levels on a wide test population, properly including the physiological variability in wrist morphology and circumference; a wider test population should be involved also to collect data better fulfilling the normality condition. This statement is supported by the results that show an increase of force at every tightening level. Further studies can be conducted by including an inertial sensor (e.g., 3-axis accelerometer) to identify the potential motion artefacts corrupting the PPG measurement and, consequently, to improve the physiological monitoring. Moreover, it would be interesting to compare HR values obtained by means of PPG sensors with those measured by a gold-standard instrument (e.g., electrocardiograph), evaluating the different band tightening levels, in order to verify how the contact pressure influences the reliability of the wearable device measurement, hence contributing to provide a more accurate understanding of healthy subjects' and patients' conditions.

References

1. Telemetry viewer. http://www.farrellf.com/TelemetryViewer/
2. Alsulami, M.H., Almuayqil, S.N., Atkins, A.S.: A comparison between heart-rate monitoring smart devices for ambient assisted living. J. Ambient Intell. Hum. Comput. 1–12 (2021). https://doi.org/10.1007/s12652-021-03025-y
3. Belmonte-Fernández, Ó., Puertas-Cabedo, A., Torres-Sospedra, J., Montoliu-Colás, R., Trilles-Oliver, S.: An indoor positioning system based on wearables for ambient-assisted living. Sensors 17(12), 36 (2016)
4. Bhagat, Y.A., Das, K., Bui, T.: Show me the SO2: real-time led oximetry display on multimodal wearable devices. In: Cullum, B.M., Kiehl, D., McLamore, E.S. (eds.) Smart Biomedical and Physiological Sensor Technology XVIII. vol. 11757, pp. 15–20. International Society for Optics and Photonics, SPIE (2021), https://doi.org/10.1117/12.2588173
5. Can, Y.S., Ersoy, C.: Privacy-preserving federated deep learning for wearable IoT-based biomedical monitoring. ACM Trans. Internet Technol. 21(1), 1–7 (2021)
6. Casaccia, S., Revel, G., Cosoli, G., Scalise, L.: Assessment of domestic well-being: from perception to measurement. IEEE Int. Instr. Measure Mag. 24(6), 58–67 (2021)
7. Casaccia, S., et al.: Measurement of users' well-being through domotic sensors and machine learning algorithms. IEEE Sens. J. 20(14), 8029–8038 (2020)
8. Casaccia, S., Revel, G.M., Scalise, L., Cucchieri, G., Rossi, L.: Smartwatches selection: market analysis and metrological characterization on the measurement of number of steps. In: 2021 IEEE International Symposium on Medical Measurements and Applications (MeMeA), pp. 1–5 (2021). https://doi.org/10.1109/MeMeA52024.2021.9478770

9. Cosoli, G., Iadarola, G., Poli, A., Spinsante, S.: Learning classifiers for analysis of blood volume pulse signals in IoT-enabled systems. In: IEEE MetroInd4.0 & IoT, Virtual Conference (2021). https://www.metroind40iot.org/

10. Cosoli, G., Scalise, L., Poli, A., Spinsante, S.: Wearable devices as a valid support for diagnostic excellence: lessons from a pandemic going forward. Health Technol. **11**(3), 673–675 (2021)

11. Cosoli, G., Spinsante, S., Scalise, L.: Wrist-worn and chest-strap wearable devices: systematic review on accuracy and metrological characteristics. Measurement p. 107789 (2020), https://linkinghub.elsevier.com/retrieve/pii/S0263224120303274

12. Cosoli, G., Spinsante, S., Scardulla, F., D'Acquisto, L., Scalise, L.: Wireless ECG and cardiac monitoring systems: State of the art, available commercial devices and useful electronic components. Measure. J. Int. Measure. Confed. **177**, 109243 (2021)

13. Culić, A., Nižetić, S., Šolić, P., Perković, T., Čongradac, V.: Smart monitoring technologies for personal thermal comfort: a review. J. Cleaner Prod. **312**, 127685 (2021)

14. Drummond, G.B., Fischer, D., Lees, M., Bates, A., Mann, J., Arvind, D.: Classifying signals from a wearable accelerometer device to measure respiratory rate. ERJ Open Res. **7**(2) (2021). https://doi.org/10.1183/23120541.00681-2020

15. Düking, P., Giessing, L., Frenkel, M.O., Koehler, K., Holmberg, H.C., Sperlich, B.: Wrist-worn wearables for monitoring heart rate and energy expenditure while sitting or performing light-to-vigorous physical activity: Validation study. JMIR Mhealth Uhealth **8**(5), e16716 (2020)

16. Haghi, M., Danyali, S., Ayasseh, S., Wang, J., Aazami, R., Deserno, T.M.: Wearable devices in health monitoring from the environmental towards multiple domains: A survey. Sensors **21**(6) (2021). https://doi.org/10.3390/s21062130. Article Number 2130

17. Hao, Y., Ma, X.K., Zhu, Z., Cao, Z.B.: Validity of wrist-wearable activity devices for estimating physical activity in adolescents: comparative study. JMIR Mhealth Uhealth **9**(1), e18320 (2021)

18. Hayashi, M., Yoshikawa, H., Uchiyama, A., Higashino, T.: Preliminary investigation on band tightness estimation of wrist-worn devices using inertial sensors. In: O'Hare, G.M.P., O'Grady, M.J., O'Donoghue, J., Henn, P. (eds.) MobiHealth 2019. LNICST, vol. 320, pp. 256–266. Springer, Cham (2020). https://doi.org/10.1007/978-3-030-49289-2_20

19. Hinde, K., White, G., Armstrong, N.: Wearable devices suitable for monitoring twenty four hour heart rate variability in military populations. Sensors **21**(4), 1061 (2021)

20. Iqbal, S.M., Mahgoub, I., Du, E., Leavitt, M.A., Asghar, W.: Advances in healthcare wearable devices. NPJ Flexible Electronics **5**(1), 1–14 (2021)

21. Jin, N., Zhang, X., Hou, Z., Sanz-Prieto, I., Mohammed, B.S.: Iot based psychological and physical stress evaluation in sportsmen using heart rate variability. Aggression and Violent Behavior 101587 (2021)

22. Kwon, S., Kim, H., Yeo, W.H.: Recent advances in wearable sensors and portable electronics for sleep monitoring. iScience **24**(5), 102461 (2021)

23. Leonidis, A., et al.: Improving stress management and sleep hygiene in intelligent homes. Sensors **21**(7), 2398 (2021)

24. Mahloko, L., Adebesin, F.: A systematic literature review of the factors that influence the accuracy of consumer wearable health device data. In: Hattingh, M., Matthee, M., Smuts, H., Pappas, I., Dwivedi, Y.K., Mäntymäki, M. (eds.) I3E 2020. LNCS, vol. 12067, pp. 96–107. Springer, Cham (2020). https://doi.org/10.1007/978-3-030-45002-1_9

25. Moraes, J.L., et al.: Advances in photopletysmography signal analysis for biomedical applications. Sensors 18(6), 1894 (2018)

26. Morresi, N., Casaccia, S., Sorcinelli, M., Arnesano, M., Uriarte, A., Torrens-Galdiz, J.I., Revel, G.M.: Sensing physiological and environmental quantities to measure human thermal comfort through machine learning techniques. IEEE Sens. J. 21(10), 12322–12337 (2021)

27. Mühlen, J.M., et al.: Recommendations for determining the validity of consumer wearable heart rate devices: expert statement and checklist of the INTERLIVE network. British J. Sports Med. 55(14), 767–779 (2021)

28. Poli, A., Cosoli, G., Scalise, L., Spinsante, S.: Impact of wearable measurement properties and data quality on ADLs classification accuracy. IEEE Sens J. 21(13), 14221–14231 (2021)

29. Přibil, J., Přibilová, A., Frollo, I.: Comparative measurement of the ppg signal on different human body positions by sensors working in reflection and transmission modes. In: Engineering Proceedings vol. 2, no. 1, p. 69 (2020)

30. Regalia, G., Onorati, F., Lai, M., Caborni, C., Picard, R.W.: Multimodal wrist-worn devices for seizure detection and advancing research: focus on the empatica wristbands. Epilepsy Res. 153, 79–82 (2019)

31. Scalise, L., Cosoli, G.: Wearables for health and fitness: Measurement characteristics and accuracy. In: I2MTC 2018–2018 IEEE International Instrumentation and Measurement Technology Conference: Discovering New Horizons in Instrumentation and Measurement, Proceedings, pp. 1–6. Institute of Electrical and Electronics Engineers Inc. (2018).https://doi.org/10.1109/I2MTC.2018.8409635

32. Scardulla, F., D'acquisto, L., Colombarini, R., Hu, S., Pasta, S., Bellavia, D.: A study on the effect of contact pressure during physical activity on photoplethysmographic heart rate measurements. Sensors (Switzerland) 20(18), 1–15 (2020)

33. Stojanović, R., Škraba, A., Lutovac, B.: A headset like wearable device to track covid-19 symptoms. In: 2020 9th Mediterranean Conference on Embedded Computing (MECO), pp. 1–4 (2020). https://doi.org/10.1109/MECO49872.2020.9134211

34. Tamura, T., Maeda, Y., Sekine, M., Yoshida, M.: Wearable photoplethysmographic sensors-past and present. Electronics 3(2), 282–302 (2014)

35. Teixeira, E., et al.: Wearable devices for physical activity and healthcare monitoring in elderly people: a critical review. Geriatrics 6(2), 38 (2021)

36. Zhang, Y., et al.: Relationship between major depression symptom severity and sleep collected using a wristband wearable device: multicenter longitudinal observational study. JMIR mHealth and uHealth 9, e24604 (2021)

37. Zhao, J., Li, G.: Study on real-time wearable sport health device based on body sensor networks. Comput. Commun. 154, 40–47 (2020)

Author Index

Printed in the United States
by Baker & Taylor Publisher Services